# Teaching in Your Office

## Second Edition

## Books in the ACP Teaching Medicine Series

**Theory and Practice of Teaching Medicine**
Jack Ende, MD, MACP
*Editor*

**Methods for Teaching Medicine**
Kelley M. Skeff, MD, PhD, MACP
Georgette A. Stratos, PhD
*Editors*

**Teaching in Your Office, A Guide to Instructing Medical Students and Residents, Second Edition**
Patrick C. Alguire, MD, FACP
Dawn E. DeWitt, MD, MSc, FACP
Linda E. Pinsky, MD, FACP
Gary S. Ferenchick, MD, FACP
*Editors*

**Teaching in the Hospital**
Jeff Wiese, MD, FACP
*Editor*

**Mentoring in Academic Medicine**
Holly J. Humphrey, MD, MACP
*Editor*

**Leadership Careers in Medical Education**
Louis Pangaro, MD, MACP
*Editor*

# Teaching Medicine Series

**Jack Ende, MD, MACP**
Series Editor

# Teaching in Your Office

## A Guide to Instructing Medical Students and Residents, Second Edition

**Patrick C. Alguire, MD, FACP**
**Dawn E. DeWitt, MD, MSc, FACP**
**Linda E. Pinsky, MD, FACP**
**Gary S. Ferenchick, MD, FACP**
Editors

ACP Press
American College of Physicians • Philadelphia, Pennsylvania

Associate Publisher and Manager, Books Publishing: Tom Hartman
Production Supervisor: Allan S. Kleinberg
Senior Editor: Karen C. Nolan
Editorial Coordinator: Angela Gabella
Text Design and Composition: Michael E. Ripca
Cover Design: Kate Nichols
Indexer: Kathleen Patterson

Printed in the United States of America
Printing/binding by Versa Press

Library of Congress Cataloging-in-Publication Data

Teaching in your office: a guide to instructing medical students and
residents / Patrick C. Alguire ... [et al.]. — 2nd ed.
    p. ; cm.
    Includes bibliographical references and index.
    ISBN 978-1-934465-02-8
    1. Medicine—Stude and teaching (Preceptorship)—United States.
    2. Ambulatory medical care—Study and teaching—United States.
    3. Medicine—Study and teaching (Residency)—United States. I. Alguire,
    Patrick C. (Patrick Craig), 1950- II. American College of Physicians (2003– )
    [DNLM: 1. Education, Medical—methods. 2. Preceptorship—methods. 3.
    Teaching—methods. W 18 T2515 2008]

R837.P74L43 2008
610.71'173—dc22
                        2007050839

15  16  17  18  19  20  /  10  9  8  7  6

# Contents

Visit www.acponline.org/acp_press/teaching
for additional information.

# About the *Teaching Medicine* Series

This book series, *Teaching Medicine*, represents a major initiative from the American College of Physicians. It is intended for College members but also for the profession as a whole. Internists, family physicians, subspecialists, surgical colleagues, nurse practitioners, and physician assistants—indeed, anyone involved with medical education—should find this book series useful as they pursue one of the greatest privileges of the profession: the opportunity to teach and make a difference in the lives of learners and their patients. The series is composed of six books:

- *Theory and Practice of Teaching Medicine*, edited by me, considers how medical learners learn (how to be doctors), how medical teachers teach, and how they (the teachers) might learn to teach better.

- *Methods for Teaching Medicine*, edited by Kelley M. Skeff and Georgette A. Stratos, builds on this foundation but focuses on the actual methods that medical teachers use. This book explores the full range of techniques that encourage learning within groups. The authors present a conceptual framework and guiding perspectives for understanding teaching; the factors that support choices for particular teaching methods (such as lecturing vs. small group discussion); and practical advice for preceptors, attendings, lecturers, discussion leaders, workshop leaders, and, finally, course directors charged with running programs for continuing medical education.

- *Teaching in Your Office*, edited by Patrick C. Alguire, Dawn E. DeWitt, Linda E. Pinsky, and Gary S. Ferenchick, will be familiar to many teaching internists. It has been reissued as part of this series. This book remains the office-based preceptor's single most useful resource for preparing to receive medical students and residents into an ambulatory practice setting or, among those already engaged in office-based teaching, for learning how to do it even better.

- *Teaching in the Hospital* is edited by Jeff Wiese and considers the challenges and rewards of teaching in that particular setting. Hospitalists as well as more traditional internists who attend on the inpatient service will be interested in the insightful advice that this book provides. This advice focuses not only on how to conduct rounds and encourage learning among students and house officers but also on how to frame and orient the content of rounds for some of the more frequently encountered inpatient conditions.

- *Mentoring in Academic Medicine,* edited by Holly J. Humphrey, considers professional development across the continuum of medical education, from issues pertaining to students to residents to faculty themselves, as well as issues pertaining to professional development of special populations. Here is where the important contributions of mentors and role models are explored in detail.

- *Leadership Careers in Medical Education* concludes this series. Edited by Louis Pangaro, this book is written for members of the medical faculty who are pursuing—or who are considering—careers as clerkship directors, residency program directors, or educational leaders of departments or medical schools, careers that require not only leadership skill but also a deep understanding of the organization and administration of internal medicine's educational enterprise. This book explores the theory and practice of educational leadership, including curricular design and evaluation; and offers insightful profiles of many of internal medicine's most prominent leaders.

*Jack Ende, MD, MACP*
*Philadelphia, 2010*

# Preface

The second edition of *Teaching in Your Office* continues our mission of providing needed resources for physicians interested in improving their skills in office-based teaching. Teaching, particularly in the ambulatory setting, takes place in a fast-paced, chaotic environment where few of us were actually trained and fewer still are prepared to take on a teaching role. Office-based physicians often believe that they do not have the time to teach or the teaching skills to do so. Many physicians who teach have never observed others teach or received feedback on their own teaching skills. Consequently, preceptors consider the opportunity for self-improvement to be limited.

This book intends to help office-based physicians improve their own teaching while maintaining the efficiency of their practice. It is designed to allow busy clinicians to identify and read only those chapters that address their specific needs. In other words, *Teaching in Your Office* does not need to be read cover to cover; rather, it can be read selectively. The second edition is enriched with additional references, inclusion of information on the "new competencies," more innovative teaching tips, a new chapter on teaching procedural skills, and a greatly expanded chapter on learner feedback and evaluation. Additionally, the appendices have been reorganized to be more accessible and intuitive. Finally, the second edition has been enhanced with an online collection (www.acponline.org/acp_press/teaching_in_your_office) of additional educational tools, faculty development resources, and an electronic teaching encounter form for mobile devices (smart phones, PDAs) or your personal computer to help you record and remember interactions with your learners. This information may be helpful when completing the learner's final evaluation. The following paragraphs describe each of the major sections and who would benefit from reading them.

## ❖ Making an Informed Decision About Precepting (Chapter 1)

This chapter is for physicians who have never taught in their offices and want to know why they should teach, what teaching entails, and its potential costs and benefits. This section also describes the "pre-requisites" for office-based teaching and where to turn for help in improving teaching skills.

## ❖ The Curriculum (Chapter 2)

This chapter describes what the student or resident is expected to accomplish when participating in an office-based teaching experience. It is useful for physicians who teach, but who have not been told what to teach, clinicians who have been asked to help plan an office-based curriculum, and to learn about the ACGME six core competency areas including how they can be taught and evaluated in the office setting.

## ❖ Getting Ready to Teach (Chapter 3)

This chapter describes how to prepare the office and staff for teaching, conduct a learner orientation, schedule patients when a learner is present, and prepare learning activities for the novice learner. It also addresses how to document a patient visit for billing purposes when a learner has participated in patient care. This section will be particularly helpful for new teachers or teachers trying to improve their efficiency.

## ❖ Teaching Skills and Organizational Techniques for Office-Based Teaching (Chapter 4)

This chapter provides a definition of meaningful patient responsibility, describes the characteristics of effective teachers, provides tips on how to help learners organize their visit with the patient, and advice on how to select appropriate patients for learners. Novices and experienced teachers will benefit from this chapter.

## ❖ Case-Based Learning (Chapter 5)

This chapter defines case-based learning and provides descriptions of seven different case-based learning models for office-based teaching, the pitfalls of case-based learning, and how to conclude the day. All preceptors will benefit from reading this section.

### ❖ Ways to Be More Efficient When Teaching (Chapter 6)

This chapter presents tips on how to teach efficiently (getting more done in less time) yet effectively. The contents of this section were set aside specifically for preceptors wishing to minimize the effect of office-based teaching on productivity or the length of their day; however, it contains useful teaching suggestions for all preceptors, regardless of concerns about efficiency.

### ❖ Teaching Procedures in the Office (Chapter 7)

This new chapter describes a method of teaching procedures to learners including the creation of learning objectives, how to break a skill down into its component parts and create a skill checklist, introducing a skill, and a description and pointers on the various phases of practice. An example of teaching a common office procedure is provided to illustrate the teaching points.

### ❖ Learner Feedback and Evaluation (Chapter 8)

This greatly expanded section describes how to give effective feedback to learners, evaluate a learner, give feedback efficiently, and how to use simple yet valid evaluation strategies. Additionally, new information on how to evaluate case presentations is included. This section concludes with advice on how to avoid common evaluation errors and how to conduct the final evaluation session. All preceptors should read the sections on feedback, whereas preceptors who must provide a formal evaluation of the learner to the sponsoring institution should review the section on evaluation.

### ❖ Preceptor Evaluation and Teaching Improvement (Chapter 9)

This chapter provides information on how preceptors are evaluated by their learners, examples of how this information is used by the sponsoring institution, tips on how to continue the process of improving teaching skills, and new information on reflection as it pertains to improving teaching skills.

### ❖ Tools, Summaries and Checklists, Resources (Appendices A, B, and C)

Collected in the back of the book are summaries of the major points described in the text, useful data collection and organizational tools, and resources intended to make the job of teaching easier and more efficient. Some experienced teachers may prefer to read only this section as a "refresher," but most preceptors will find the material in this section helpful both as a summary and as a source of practical teaching aids.

*Patrick C. Alguire, MD*

# 1

## Making an Informed Decision About Precepting

### ❖ What Is Community-Based Teaching?

Community-based teaching is a return to the historical roots of medical education: the one-on-one teaching of students and residents by practitioners in an office setting. While community-based teachers usually do not have full-time academic appointments, exceptions to this rule are common; many full-time academic physicians who deliver care in (non-hospital) office settings are considered community-based teachers. Some community-based teachers receive a financial stipend for their participation, but many do not. What all these groups do have in common is the delivery of comprehensive, primary, or subspecialty care in an ambulatory setting to patients who recognize the teacher as their personal physician. Community-based teaching establishes an environment of "educational intimacy," consisting of one teacher, one learner, and one patient: a place where role modeling, assessment, feedback, and evaluation are maximized for the benefit of the learner (1).

## ❖ Why Is Community-Based Teaching Needed?

Teaching institutions need community-based practitioners who are willing to teach in their offices. Decreasing numbers of inpatients with shorter lengths of stay and higher illness intensity and the growing mismatch between the educational content and clinical practice of medicine have resulted in a greater emphasis on ambulatory training. One study showed that only 30% of patients in teaching hospitals were appropriate, available in their rooms, and willing to see medical students (2). Ambulatory settings provide the best opportunity to learn about common outpatient problems, chronic disease management, screening, health maintenance, doctor-patient relationships, and some psychosocial aspects of care (3,4).

However, not all ambulatory settings are equal. The traditional ambulatory environment is the academic medical center or the hospital-based clinic. In this setting, a single faculty member may supervise three to five learners caring for patients who may not recognize the supervising faculty as their "personal physician." In contrast, the community-based office can provide an outstanding educational environment with one-to-one mentoring. Also, the close relationships that develop between physicians and learners provide an opportunity for role modeling that cannot be reproduced in other settings.

Community-based teaching is rapidly becoming the standard for medical student and resident education. In 1984, only 7% of residency programs offered office assignments for internal medicine residents (5); by 2001, 94% of medical schools used community preceptors as clinical teachers, especially in ambulatory settings (6). Additionally, 84% of internal medicine clerkships nationwide require an ambulatory experience as part of their basic educational experience (2002 CDIM Survey Results [on-line] access at www.im.org/AAIM/Data/Docs/ 2002CDIMSurvey. ppt on 18 July 2007).

Among programs offering community-based training, ambulatory education accounts for more than 10% of training time for upper-level residents (Unpublished data, American College of Physicians).

However, this success has created problems. Office-based preceptors are a scarce commodity (7). Recruiting qualified preceptors is difficult, and it may be getting harder (8). A preponderance of schools report that preceptors are less likely to volunteer because of economic pressures in their offices that force them to become more efficient. There is increasing competition between medical schools, residency programs, and training programs for physician assistants and nurse practitioners for access to preceptors (8).

Finally, as the U.S. and other countries increase medical student numbers to address doctor shortages, ambulatory community-based settings are viewed as an ideal venue for education. Thus, there is an urgent need to attract more physicians to community-based teaching programs to provide excellent training opportunities for future doctors (9).

### ❖ How Good Is the Training in Community Offices?

Office-based teaching offers certain educational experiences that are more representative of "real world" medicine compared with the traditional hospital-based clinic. Students in community-based settings see more patients, are exposed to a wider variety of patient problems, provide more acute care, evaluate more patients in the emergency department, and perform more procedures than students assigned to traditional hospital-based clinics. Furthermore, compared with students in traditional clinic settings, students in community settings are more likely to be supervised closely, to see patients in follow-up, to discuss the patient's case with a preceptor, to witness the preceptor delivering care, and to rate their experiences highly (4,10-14).

Training in ambulatory settings away from the academic medical center must facilitate mastery of the required medical content to a level equal to that which is achieved in the academic medical center. Data to support or refute equivalence of the training at these sites are difficult to collect. The published studies to date show no evidence of decreased mastery of core content when students are assigned on a part-time basis to community offices compared with students who receive all of their training at academic medical centers. Although most of these studies were not randomized —which decreases their validity—the results of these nonrandomized studies are encouraging. Compared with students at academic medical centers (including hospital-based ambulatory clinics), students assigned on a part-time basis to community offices have similar scores on end-of-rotation evaluation exercises, including oral examinations, practical clinical examinations, and the National Board of Medical Examiners subject examination.

Furthermore, students spending part of their training time in a practitioner's office have similar clerkship grades and number of honors grades compared with students who receive all of their training at the academic medical center (10,15,16). On the other hand, students trained part-time in office settings may have more opportunity for continuity of care and have improved skills in clinical diagnosis, laboratory interpretation, doctor-patient relationships, and communication skills compared with their peers trained entirely in the academic medical center (4,15-20). Learners are more likely to care for patients with chronic conditions in community-based practices and observe their preceptor conduct histories and physical examinations (20). Student satisfaction concerning the overall educational value, patient mix, workload, faculty interest, and involvement in patient care has been noted to be higher as a result of training in a community site. The bottom line is that existing studies find no meaningful educational difference in student competencies as a result of part-time community training (21).

Initial fears that the office-based experience does not sufficiently involve students in patient care also seem to be unfounded. Students report that they are just as involved in patient care as when they were in the hospital, i.e., they have adequate supervision, have sufficient learning time, see a wider variety of patients and problems, and perform minimal "scut" work (17). Finally, residents rate their quality of supervision in private offices as being better than what they experienced in institutional clinics or health-maintenance organizations (HMOs) (22). Existing data suggests that preceptors rather than sites make the greatest difference in successful ambulatory care experiences for learners (23). Confidence in community-based teaching may be best exemplified by the Australian "Rural Clinical School" program, which now provides community-based training for at least one clinical year for 25% of all "metropolitan teaching hospital"–based students (24). In summary, the available data suggest that office-based training seems more enjoyable, varied, active, and supervised than traditional training.

## ❖ What Do Community-Based Practitioners Have to Offer Learners and Why Is It So Valuable?

Many physicians are reluctant to participate in community-based teaching because they believe they lack the time and talent to "teach." Many community physicians equate teaching with giving "lectures." In fact, this is not what learners, medical schools, and residency programs want from preceptors; they want exposure to practical skills. In this light, most community-based physicians *can* teach efficiently and effectively. In one study, students identified critical learning events in office-based settings. Typically, important teaching moments lasted less than five minutes, focused on problems (rather than on an abstract review of a topic), and had a practical outcome. The single most important learning event identified by students was observing an experienced physician interacting with a patient. This is not to suggest that the entire experience should be observational. On the contrary, students and residents crave the opportunity to actively deliver care (i.e., first seeing the patient alone, then with the preceptor), but the opportunity to watch an expert deal with a difficult problem is highly valued. Other highly rated learning events include improving communication and clinical skills (17,25), validating the learners' impression or plan, and verifying a physical finding (26). These are important abilities that preceptors have in abundance, and they require little in the way of preparation to be presented effectively to the learner.

The take-home message to office-based preceptors is that students who participate in office-based experiences value learning the process of care as much as, or possibly more than, mastering core content. Students and residents crave the real-world experience of caring for patients, which office-based practitioners can provide.

## ❖ What Is the Preceptor's Role?

Preceptors are responsible for learner orientation, including setting and clarifying expectations; providing learning opportunities and demonstrating basic ambulatory medicine knowledge and skills; assessing learner performance and providing corrective feedback; and demonstrating professionalism and enthusiasm for medicine. Trainees consider preceptors excellent teachers if they love what they do, are enthusiastic about their career and convey that excitement to their learners. The most powerful influence on a novice learner is a preceptor who provides a positive role model of the doctor-patient relationship (23). Just as importantly, preceptors should engage the office staff to develop an excellent learning environment. Explaining to staff and colleagues what you want the learner to do and see may include everything from recruiting patients to how the learner spends time with other staff in the office.

## ❖ What Do Learners Want from a Community-Based Teaching Experience?

The message from the learners is consistent and clear: they want the opportunity to practice patient management, basic data collection, and interpretation skills on the wide variety of patients typically seen in the office setting. They desire feedback on their performance and a role model to emulate. To students, the preceptor's characteristics are the most important factor defining a successful office-based experience; of these, the most highly rated is the preceptor's ability to promote student independence (27). Most often this is accomplished by giving the student increasing patient care responsibility. Other highly favored characteristics include the preceptor's willingness to allow the student 1) to practice technical and problem-solving skills, 2) to show enthusiasm and interest in patients, and 3) to be actively involved in the learning process. The willingness of a preceptor to act as a mentor and to advise the student is also highly valued (17,25,27). While there is a striking degree of similarity in what is valued by learners, differences do exist, particularly among learners at different levels. Preceptor interaction is most valued by medical students in contrast to residents who value issues pertaining to patient logistics and office flow and practice management (28).

Although the characteristics of the office itself are important to learners, they are secondary to preceptor characteristics. Valued office characteristics include having many different preceptors available, a variety of patient problems, and a range of patient ages (27).

The areas that provide the most difficulty for students are learning to work within the time constraints of the office setting, performing a focused examination, and learning to rely on data-gathering skills and problem-solving abilities rather than on imaging and laboratory tests (29). Preceptors, by virtue of their everyday experience, can provide valuable tips and direction to help learners develop these skill sets. Residents value the opportunity to discuss differential diagnosis and management issues, and they appreciate close supervision, feedback, and the opportunity to practice and improve clinical and procedural skills (30).

## ❖ How Do Learners Rate the Community Experience and Preceptors?

Students and residents value their time with community preceptors and recognize the unique contributions the office-based experience brings to their training. Student evaluations rate volunteer preceptors as highly as they do full-time faculty (31), and even higher in their showing interest (13). When students were asked to compare their community-based experience with other clerkships, the office experience was seen as contributing most to their acquisition of improved clinical and communication skills and improved awareness of issues relating to cost-effectiveness. Comparing their community-based experiences with traditional clerkship rotations, students reported learning as much about disease pattern recognition and the ability to generate a differential diagnosis and actually learned *more* about managing chronic medical and psychosocial problems and evaluating patients' "hidden agenda" items (17,25,32).

## ❖ What Are the Concerns of Practitioners Involved in Community-Based Teaching?

Practitioners involved in office-based teaching frequently voice concerns over potential costs and time required for teaching (3,33). Other concerns include 1) poor matching of student with preceptor; 2) dealing with potential teacher-learner conflicts, poorly motivated learners, and inappropriate learner behavior; and 3) the effect of office teaching on patient satisfaction (34). Preceptors are concerned about their ability to provide a good educational experience for the learner and their lack of resources (e.g., textbooks, computers) to support teaching (34). Additionally preceptors are more comfortable in their abilities as clinicians than as teachers. For example, behaviors associated with clinical practice (e.g., confirming clinical findings) occur more confidently than teaching behaviors that enhance learning such as giving feedback to students, particularly if it is negative (23). Preceptors also want to be assured that the institution will cover the learner's malpractice insurance, which it will. The following paragraphs address these important concerns and provide physicians with the necessary information to help them decide whether or not to be an office-based preceptor.

## ❖ What Are Some of the Costs Associated with Community-Based Teaching?

The two most commonly cited costs of office-based teaching are preceptor time and lost billings. Most studies involving students show an increase in the workday of 45 minutes to an hour for each half-day teaching session (33,35). Results of studies assessing productivity vary from showing no loss of productivity or revenue (but a longer workday) to seeing one less patient each half-day session, corresponding to reduced charges of $55 to $60 (35-40). A financial model based on prospective log data from both students and preceptors in rural "general"(family) practice showed that students contributed to productivity without any impact on patient satisfaction if they were based in a practice for more than 5 months (41). In another study, two thirds of physicians reported no loss of income (33). The presence of a student does not seem to be associated with increased "hidden costs" (e.g., more laboratory tests, prescriptions, or referrals to other physicians), an important consideration in a "managed" health care system (42).

Other studies have documented that the time actually spent in direct contact with a student is just over three hours for each half-day session, considerably more than the time documented for inpatient teaching (43). Approximately 30 minutes to an hour of the contact time is spent alone with the student; the balance is with the student and patient (23,39,43,44). Studies have not been reported for residents participating in office-based teaching; however, it is likely that the results would be similar. Although residents are more clinically capable, most practitioners see residents' patients (briefly) to maintain the doctor-patient relationship and to justify billing.

### ❖ What Are the Practitioner Benefits of Community-Based Teaching?

Community preceptors repeatedly report that precepting makes them enjoy clinical practice more (33,39,45,46). Most preceptors report a fulfilling sense of "giving something back" to medicine (47). For example, demonstration projects have identified that satisfaction in being involved in training of the next generation of physicians, pride in contributing to the growth of students' knowledge and skills, and being seen by students as a role model were important "affective benefits" experienced by community-based teachers (48). Others have commented on a decreased sense of professional isolation and the rewards of sharing knowledge and a vision of the specialty with the learner (46). Enhanced respect from patients and colleagues, along with increased staff satisfaction has been identified as other "affective benefits" by community-based teachers (45). Keeping up with the medical literature and reviewing basic sciences and clinical skills also are frequently reported as benefits of community-based teaching (39,46,47,49). Some physicians and institutions use precepting as a method to recruit newly graduated residents as employees or partners (33,50). There is even a suggestion that office-based education results in increased time spent in patient education, a value-added benefit of teaching that is reaped by patients (45). One potential economic windfall is a higher capitation rate for participating physicians negotiated in their behalf by the training institution. A 1% increase in the capitation rate has been negotiated by medical schools, which is a tangible reward despite its tendency to be a rather small sum of money (50). This strategy can be employed by most teaching institutions for their office preceptors.

## ❖ What Are the Most Commonly Offered Rewards for Community-Based Teaching?

Most preceptors are rewarded for their participation in office-based teaching programs, but typically the reward is not financial. Just over half of medical schools provide clinical appointments to volunteer faculty, but only 15% provide a financial stipend (11,36).

Although it is likely that practitioners would appreciate financial reimbursement for their efforts, most acknowledge that institutions cannot begin to pay what their teaching is worth. Nevertheless, practitioners are consistent in their desire to have their contribution recognized in some meaningful way (11,35,36,46,49,51). The value of the reward to the practitioner differs according to the practice type and location (51). (For a more detailed description, see Commonly Offered Rewards for Precepting in Appendix C on page 172).

## ❖ How Do Patients React to Office-Based Teaching?

One reason physicians may not participate in office-based teaching is their concerns about quality of care and patient satisfaction when a learner is in the office (7). To address these concerns, studies have been performed in both staff-model HMOs and traditional office practices. In the HMO setting, over 90% of the participating physicians and their patients indicated that quality of care and patient satisfaction were unaffected by the presence of students (39). Another survey found that 83% of patients interacting with first year medical students "enjoyed" their interaction (52). Similar results can be found in surveys of physicians in private practice and by questioning their patients directly (42,53). Many patients report enjoying the extra attention they receive from the learner and are impressed that their personal physician is involved in training students and residents (54). Negative reactions to students are uncommon even around issues of repeating parts of the examination performed by the student, discussing personal issues in front of a student, or extending the length of the visit (54,55). Despite the rarity of negative experiences, it remains the prerogative of the patient to decline participation in office-based teaching, and consent always should be obtained before involving a student or resident in their care. When known well in advance, many preceptors rely on their front office staff to alert patients that a student will be in the office and to obtain their consent when scheduling the appointment.

## ❖ What Are the Prerequisites for Precepting?

Most institutions that need community-based preceptors do not require previous teaching experience as a pre-requisite. In fact, few full-time academic faculty have ever been taught how to teach. Nevertheless, faculty-development programs can be a helpful resource to improve teaching effectiveness and are recommended. In the interim, most community physicians can provide useful educational experiences to learners without formal training in teaching. Community preceptors have daily experience in teaching with their patients and the skills they have developed are valuable for teaching learners. As Charles Griffith has written about teaching effectiveness, "… the best teachers do not necessarily impart more factual knowledge (facts which may be obsolete in a few years), but rather they engender a learning climate that makes learning fun, enjoyable and exciting" (56). Keep in mind that what most learners want out of the experience is the opportunity to observe problems common to the ambulatory setting and then to practice treating them. They also desire feedback on their performance. Learners in the ambulatory setting are less interested in lectures and more interested in the "how to" process. Learners crave "real world" experiences with role models that care for patients. It is also important to understand that learners don't want a "shadowing" experience, i.e., following a preceptor from patient to patient simply observing the care that is given. Essentially, learners want meaningful and independent responsibility. Initially, this means having opportunities to see the patient alone. After this step, there are many teaching strategies that detail how to teach and provide care in ways that are efficient and satisfying to both the learner and the patient (see Chapter 5).

## ❖ Are There Courses to Improve Your Teaching?

For those interested in improving their teaching skills, this book helps lay a foundation; however, as with any learning situation, being observed and receiving feedback is probably the most effective method to improve your teaching. Many medical schools and residency programs provide workshops designed to improve teaching, and they will be happy to involve you. Some teaching workshops are offered at national meetings.

Due to their timing, duration, or location, faculty-development workshops may not be a feasible option for all physicians. To meet the needs of these preceptors, some teaching programs have put their faculty-development programs on the Internet or on CD-ROM, or they have created instructional videotapes and companion texts. Most of these programs are free or available for a modest price. For a listing of available faculty-development workshops or resources near you, call the Department of Continuing Medical Education at your local hospital, medical school, or professional society. Faculty development resources can also be identified by searching the Internet. On your web browser enter the search terms "Faculty Development" AND >your specialty<. For example, to search for faculty development resources in internal medicine enter "faculty development" AND "internal medicine." (For more information, see Faculty Development Resources for Preceptors in Appendix C on page 173, and visit the electronic enhancements of this book at www.acponline.org/acp_press/ teaching_in_your_office.)

# REFERENCES

1. **Irby DM.** Teaching and learning in ambulatory care settings: a thematic review of the literature. Acad Med. 1995;70:898-931.
2. **Olson LG, Hill SR, Newby DA.** Barriers to student access to patients in a group of teaching hospitals. Med J Aust. 2005;183:461-3.
3. **Woolliscroft JO, Schwenk TL.** Teaching and learning in the ambulatory setting. Acad Med. 1989;64:644-8.
4. **Butterfield PS, Libertin AG.** Learning outcomes of an ambulatory care rotation in internal medicine for junior medical students. J Gen Intern Med. 1993;8:189-92.
5. **Napodano RJ, Schuster BL, Krackov SK, et al.** Use of private offices in education of residents in internal medicine. Arch Intern Med. 1984;144:303-5.
6. **Walling AD, Sutton LD, Gold J.** Administrative relationships between medical schools and community preceptors. Acad Med. 2001;76:184-7.
7. **Levinsky NG.** A survey of changes in the proportions of ambulatory training in internal medicine and residencies from 1986-1987 and from 1996-1997. Acad Med. 1998;73:1114-5.
8. **Barzansky B, Jonas HS, Etzel SI.** Educational programs in U.S. medical schools, 1998-1999. JAMA. 1999;282:840-6.
9. **DeWitt DE, Robins LS, Curtis JR, Burke W.** Primary care residency graduates' reported training needs. Acad Med. 2001;76:285.
10. **Osborn LM, Sargent JR, Williams SD.** Effects of time-in-clinic setting, and faculty supervision on the continuity clinic experience. Pediatrics. 1993;91:1089-93.
11. **Usatine RP, Lin K.** Free Internet access for community physicians. Acad Med. 1999;74:204-5.
12. **Greer T, Schneeweiss R, Baldwin LM.** A comparison of student clerkship experiences in community practices and residency-based clinics. Fam Med. 1993;25:322-6.
13. **Schwiebert LP, Ramsey CNJ, Davis A.** Comparison of volunteer and full-time faculty performance in a required third-year medicine clerkship. Teach Learn Med. 1992;4:225-32.
14. **DeWitt DE, Migeon M, LeBlond R, Carline JD, Francis L, Irby DM.** Insights from outstanding rural internal medicine residency rotations at the University of Washington. Acad Med. 2001;76:273-81.
15. **Pangaro L, Gibson K, Russell W, et al.** A prospective randomized trial of a six-week ambulatory medicine rotation. Acad Med. 1995;70:537-41.
16. **Carney PA, Ogrinc G, Harwood BG, Schiffman JS, Cochran N.** The influence of teaching setting on medical students' clinical skills development: is the academic medical center the "gold standard"? Acad Med. 2005;80:1153-8.
17. **Prislin MD, Feighny KM, Stearns JA, et al.** What students say about learning and teaching in longitudinal ambulatory primary care clerkships: a multi-institutional study. Acad Med. 1998;73:680-7.
18. **Grum CM, Case SM, Swanson DB, Woolliscroft JO.** Identifying the trees in the forest: characteristics of students who demonstrate disparity between knowledge and diagnostic pattern recognition skills. Acad Med. 1994;10(Suppl):S66-8.
19. **Papadakis M, Kagawa MK.** A randomized controlled pilot study of placing third-year medical clerks in a continuity clinic. Acad Med. 1993;68:845-7.

20. **Carney PA, Eliassen MS, Pipas CF, Genereaux SH, Nierenberg DW.** Ambulatory care education: how do academic medical centers, affiliated residency teaching sites, and community-based practices compare? Acad Med. 2004;79:69-77.

21. **Ferenchick GS, Chamberlain J, Alguire P.** Community-based teaching: defining the added value for students and preceptors. Am J Med. 2002;112:512-7.

22. **Swing SR, Vasilias J.** Internal medicine residency education in ambulatory settings. Acad Med. 1997;72:988-96.

23. **Bowen JL, Irby DM.** Assessing quality and costs of education in the ambulatory setting: a review of the literature. Acad Med. 2002;77:621-80.

24. **Maley MA, Denz-Penhey H, Lockyer-Stevens V, Murdoch JC.** Tuning medical education for rural-ready practice: designing and resourcing optimally. Med Teach. 2006;8:345-50.

25. **Epstein RM, Cole DR, Gawinski BA, et al.** How students learn from community-based preceptors. Arch Fam Med. 1998;7:149-54.

26. **Cyran EM, Albertson G, Schilling LM, Lin CT, Ware L, Steiner JF, Anderson RJ.** What do attending physicians contribute in a house officer-based ambulatory continuity clinic? J Gen Intern Med. 2006;21:435-9.

27. **Biddle WB, Riesenberg LA, Dacy PA.** Medical student's perceptions of desirable characteristics of primary care teaching sites. Fam Med. 1996;28:629-33.

28. **Schultz KW, Kirby J, Delva D, Godwin M, Verma S, Birtwhistle R, Knapper C, Seguin R.** Medical Students' and Residents' preferred site characteristics and preceptor behaviours for learning in the ambulatory setting: a cross-sectional survey. BMC Med Educ. 2004;4:12.

29. **Feltovich J, Mast TA, Soler NG.** Teaching medical students in ambulatory settings in departments of internal medicine. Acad Med. 1989;64:36-41.

30. **O'Mallery PG, Kroenke K, Ritter J, et al.** What learners and teachers value most in ambulatory educational encounters: a prospective, qualitative study. Acad Med. 1999;74:186-91.

31. **Irby DM, Gillmore GM, Ramsey PG.** Factors affecting ratings of clinical teachers by medical students and residents. J Med Educ. 1987;62:1-7.

32. **Packman CH, Krackov SK, Groff GD, Cohen J.** The Rochester practice-based experience: an experiment in medical education. Arch Intern Med. 1994;154:1253-60.

33. **Vinson DC, Paden C.** The effect of teaching medical students on private practitioner's workloads. Acad Med. 1994;69:237-8.

34. **Kollisch DO, Frasier PY, Slatt L, Storaasli M.** Community preceptors' views of a required third-year family medicine clerkship. Arch Fam Med. 1997;6:25-8.

35. **Levy BT, Gjerde CL, Albrecht LA.** The effects of precepting on and the support desired by community-based preceptors in Iowa. Acad Med. 1997;72:382-4.

36. **Vinson DC, Paden C, Devera-Sales A, et al.** Teaching medical students in community-based practices: a national survey of generalist physicians. J Fam Prac. 1997;45:487-94.

37. **Fields SA, Toffler WL, Bledsoe NM.** Impact of the presence of a third-year medical student on gross charges and patient volumes in 22 rural community practices. Acad Med. 1994;69(Suppl 10):S87-9.

38. **Kearl GW, Mainous AG.** Physicians' productivity and teaching responsibilities. Acad Med. 1993;68:166-7.

39. **Kirz HL, Larsen C.** Costs and benefits of medical student training to a health maintenance organization. JAMA. 1986;256:734-9.

40. **Foley R, Yonke A, Smith J, et al.** Recruiting and retaining volunteer community preceptors. Acad Med. 1996;71:460-3.
41. **Worley PS, Kitto P.** Hypothetical model of the financial impact of student attachments on rural general practices. Rural Remote Health. 2001;1:83. Epub 2001 Mar 2.
42. **Frank SH, Stange KC, Langa D, Workings M.** Direct observation of community-based ambulatory encounters involving medical students. JAMA. 1997;278:712-6.
43. **Ricer RE, Van Horne A, Filak AT.** Costs of preceptors' time spent teaching during a third-year family medicine outpatient rotation. Acad Med. 1997;72:547-51.
44. **Denton GD, Durning SJ, Hemmer PA, Pangaro LN.** A time and motion study of the effect of ambulatory medical students on the duration of general internal medicine clinics. Teach Learn Med. 2005;17:285-9.
45. **Grayson MS, Klein M, Lugo J, Visintainer P.** Benefits and costs to community-based physicians teaching primary care to medical students. J Gen Intern Med. 1998;13:485-8.
46. **Fulkerson PK, Wang-Cheng R.** Community-based faculty: motivations and rewards. Fam Med. 1997;29:105-7.
47. **Dodson MC.** Should private practitioners be paid for teaching? Acad Med. 1998;73:222.
48. **Ullian JA, Shore WB, First LR.** What did we learn about the impact on community-based faculty? Recommendations for recruitment, retention, and rewards. Acad Med. 2001;76:S78-85.
49. **Latessa R, Beaty N, Landis S, Colvin G, Janes C.** The Satisfaction, Motivation, and Future of Community Preceptors: The North Carolina Experience. Acad Med. 2007;82:698-703.
50. **Grayson MS, Newton DA, Klein M, Irons T.** Promoting institutional change to encourage primary care: experiences at New York Medical College and East Carolina University School of Medicine. Acad Med. 1999;74(Suppl):S9-15.
51. **Langlois JP.** Support of community-preceptors: What do they need? Fam Med. 1995;27:641-5.
52. **Usatine RP, Hodgson CS, Marshall ET, Whitman DW, Slavin SJ, Wilkes MS.** Reactions of family medicine community preceptors to teaching medical students. Fam Med. 1995;27:566-70.
53. **O'Malley PG, Omori DM, Landry FJ, Jackson J, Kroenke K.** A prospective study to assess the effect of ambulatory teaching on patient satisfaction. Acad Med. 1997;72:1015-7.
54. **Devera-Sales A, Paden C, Vinson DC.** What do family medicine patients think about medical students' participation in their health care? Acad Med. 1999;74:550-2.
55. **Gress TW, Flynn JA, Rubin HR, Simonson L, et al.** Effect of student involvement on patient perceptions of ambulatory care visits: a randomized controlled trial. J Gen Intern Med. 2002;17:420-7.
56. **Griffith CH 3rd, Georgesen JC, Wilson JF.** Six-year documentation of the association between excellent clinical teaching and improved students' examination performances. Acad Med. 2000;75:S62-4.

# 2

## The Curriculum

### ❖ Core Competencies

Medical educators are refining the mission of clinical education with emphasis on mastery of core clinical competencies. The change is being driven by mandates for improved quality, safety, and accountability in health care. The accrediting body for the U.S. residency training programs, the Accreditation Council for Graduate Medical Education (ACGME), has identified a set of competencies that all residents, regardless of specialty, should master by the end of their training. The purpose of these competencies is to set benchmarks that demonstrate successful outcomes and not simply the intention to teach these topics. Increasingly, medical schools are adopting the same core set of competencies as an organizing framework for their curricular objectives. As a preceptor, you will not be expected to teach and evaluate each of the competencies. We are presenting them to you with the expectation that awareness of the competencies allows you to see the "big picture" of medical education at the clinical level, better understand the current educational jargon, develop a deeper understanding of the institutional goals for the precepting experience, and anticipate what you may be asked to evaluate.

## Box 2-1. ACGME Core Competencies

### I. Patient Care

▶ Competency: Must be able to provide care that is compassionate, appropriate, and effective for the treatment of health problems and the promotion of health.

▶ Example: Gathers essential and accurate information about patients and carries out management plans.

### II. Medical Knowledge

▶ Competency: Must demonstrate knowledge about established and evolving biomedical, clinical, and cognate (e.g., epidemiological and social-behavioral) sciences and the application of knowledge to patient care.

▶ Example: Medical knowledge is at appropriate level and is sufficient to participate in supervised patient care.

### III. Practice-Based Learning and Improvement

▶ Competency: Must be able to investigate and evaluate their patient care practices, appraise and assimilate scientific evidence, and improve their patient care practices.

▶ Example: Uses chart audits to measure care against accepted benchmarks and performs practice-based improvement activities.

### IV. Interpersonal and Communication Skills

▶ Competency: Must be able to demonstrate interpersonal and communication skills that result in effective information exchange and teaming with patients, their families, and professional associates.

▶ Example: Uses effective listening skills and effective explanatory skills.

### V. Professionalism

▶ Competency: Must demonstrate a commitment to carrying out professional responsibilities, adhering to ethical principles, and being sensitive to a diverse patient population.

▶ Example: Demonstrates respect, compassion, and integrity and is responsive to patients' culture, age, sex and disabilities.

*continued*

**VI. Systems-Based Practice**

► Competency: Must demonstrate an awareness of and responsiveness to the larger context of health care and the ability to effectively call on system resources to provide care that is of optimal value.

► Example: Knows how to coordinate ancillary health services for patient care.

## ❖ What Are Reasonable Teaching Goals for Community-Based Teaching?

Community-based teaching sites have been used successfully to teach a wide variety of medical skills, including physical diagnosis, patient interviewing, patient education and counseling, ethics, and subspecialty medicine (1,2). Many of these areas fall naturally into one or more of the six competencies mandated by the ACGME and are more fully explained with examples. Boxes 2-1 and 2-2 highlight selected examples of office-based activities that can help learners master these skills.

The first competency, Patient Care, is the easiest for you to teach. Not unexpectedly, the office provides learners with excellent opportunities to learn how to treat common medical problems efficiently and effectively and to experience the effect that diseases have on their patients and families. The office setting provides an excellent opportunity for learners to observe, and if appropriate, practice common office procedures including: cerumen removal, incision and drainage of abscesses, interpretation of chest x-rays and electrocardiograms, administering intra-muscular (influenza) or subcutaneous (PPD) injections, knee arthrocentesis, pap smear and vaginal wet mount, skin biopsy, and venipuncture (3).

The Medical Knowledge competency is also relatively easy for most preceptors to address. Learners can to add to their clinical knowledge by reading about their patients and making short presentations at the beginning or end of the day. You can direct learners to "point of care" clinical information or evidence sources you use to manage medical problems.

## Box 2-2 Learning the ACGME Competencies

**I. Patient Care (See sections Meaningful Responsibility and Interacting Skillfully with Patients, both in Chapter 4)**

- ▶ Observing and providing acute and chronic care to patients
- ▶ Observing and performing common office-based procedures
- ▶ Observing the social, financial, and ethical aspects of medical practice
- ▶ Learning when to refer patients for specialty care

**II. Medical Knowledge (See sections Self-Directed Learning in Chapter 6 and Involving the Learner in Chapter 4)**

- ▶ Reading about patients' problems
- ▶ Making short presentations
- ▶ Using sources of evidence-based medicine to learn about patient management

**III. Problem-Based Learning and Improvement**

- ▶ Reviewing with you performance measures provided by third-party insurers
- ▶ Performing office chart audits on common medical problems and analyzing results
- ▶ Participating in office-based quality improvement efforts
- ▶ Introduction to office patient registry and electronic health record system (if available)

**IV. Interpersonal and Communication Skills (See the section Strategies for Organizing the Office Visit in Chapter 4)**

- ▶ Practicing case presentations
- ▶ Interviewing patients
- ▶ Giving patients instructions and providing patient education
- ▶ Returning patient phone calls

**V. Professionalism (See sections Role Modeling the Desired Behaviors in Chapter 4 and Reflection in Chapter 5)**

- ▶ Observing you interacting with patients, colleagues and staff
- ▶ Reflection on recent interactions with patients, colleagues, and staff

*continued*

**VI. Systems-Based Practice (See the section Service-Based Education in Chapter 6)**

- ► Observing the practice and the roles of the staff
- ► Participating with the office staff while they perform their roles
- ► Coordinating patient care
- ► Making visits with patients to ancillary services (rehabilitation, diabetic education, radiology)

Finally, learners can appreciate the natural history of disease by observing many patients with the same disease at different stages of severity.

Practice-Based Learning and Improvement sounds like a more difficult education challenge than it is and can easily be addressed by most preceptors. If your office uses a patient registry or electronic health record, show the learner how these tools generate patient reports and reminders of care. If one of your health plans provides performance measures, review them with the learner and discuss what they mean and how you intend to use them. If you are required to perform self-audits of care (for example, for your health system or recertification in your specialty), have the learner perform a limited chart audit on a well-defined health outcome (for example, mammogram utilization or hemoglobin A1c levels) and analyze the results and discuss the next steps. Additionally, practice-based learning can be reinforced by having learners identify unanswered questions as a result of their patient interactions, finding high-quality answers to these questions and sharing their learning with you (and your patients).

Learners can practice and demonstrate components of the Communication Skills competency by presenting cases to you. The office practice is also particularly well suited for teaching patient communication and negotiation skills by having the learner observe you followed by supervised practice with their assigned patients. Other readily available learning opportunities are returning patient phone calls and providing patients with follow up instructions and disease management education.

By observing you interact with patients, staff, and colleagues, learners see Professionalism in action. Asking students to reflect on what they observed, or on their own experiences, promotes professional behaviors.

Community-based teaching provides the opportunity for students and residents to learn about Systems-Based Practice including financial and reimbursement issues, team care, developing collaborative relationships between patients and health care providers, and how ancillary services are used. The learner can observe how you coordinate care for patients. Explain to your learner how each office staff member contributes to the efficient running of the office; possibly assign the learner to different staff roles in the office so they can appreciate their contributions to patient care. Learners can accompany patients to various ancillary services (for example, rehabilitation medicine, diabetic educator, and radiation therapy) to experience first hand how they are integrated into patient management.

Institutions that sponsor office-based teaching will provide, or should be encouraged to provide, you their learning objectives and goals. These should explicitly spell out the expectations for the office experience and provide benchmarks for providing feedback and evaluation of the the goals and objectives attained by the learner. However, sometimes institutional goals and objectives are voluminous and overwhelming for preceptors. If you do feel overwhelmed, you can begin to clarify these expectations by focusing on the goals that you feel are best taught and evaluated in your setting. Share the goals with the learners and ask them to participate through identifying which of the goals they need help mastering. (See the section entitled The RIME Evaluation Framework in Chapter 7 for an alternative set of simple but practical learning expectations.)

Finally, you should encourage students and residents to develop their own learning plans and goals at the beginning of the experience, with the expectation that they will be more pertinent and therefore more effective (4). (See the section Expectations in Chapter 3.)

# REFERENCES

1. **Woolliscroft JO, Schwenk TL.** Teaching and learning in the ambulatory setting. Acad Med. 1989;64:644-8.
2. **Wilkerson L, Armstrong E, Lesky L.** Faculty development for ambulatory teaching. J Gen Intern Med. 1990;5(Suppl):S44-53.
3. **DeWitt DE, Robins LS, Curtis JR, Burke W.** Primary care residency graduates' reported training needs. Acad Med. 2001;76:285.
4. **DeWitt DE, Migeon M, LeBlond R, Carline JD, Francis L, Irby DM.** Insights from outstanding rural internal medicine residency rotations at the University of Washington. Acad Med. 2001;76:273-81.

# 3

# Getting Ready to Teach

## ❖ Before the Learner Arrives

A well-designed orientation can ease a learner's transition into the office-based practice (1,2). Ideally, before the learner's arrival in your office, the training program will provide a general orientation to the experience (see Before the Learner Arrives Preparatory Checklist in Appendix B on page 148). The institution's orientation for the student will probably include the following items:

- Course syllabus with rotation goals and objectives
- Description of the learner's role in the office
- Outline of the expected teaching and learning activities
- Performance-evaluation criteria
- Recommended readings and resources
- Office-chart organization and techniques for efficient review
- Introduction to electronic health record and patient registries
- Dictation (occasionally) and charting skills
- Prescription writing
- Clinic etiquette

Approximately a week before the learner's arrival, review the information you have about the learner and the program. The medical school or residency program should provide you with basic information on the learner. Insist that institutional materials arrive far enough in advance to allow you sufficient time to plan the experience. Determine what materials and orientation the learner received before coming to the office. Review the institution's educational goals and objectives and note the level of the learner. Make sure they are compatible with what you can provide. If you have any questions, clarify them with the sponsoring institution before the learner arrives. If you have additional material about your office that the learner needs, ask the institution to forward them to the learner, especially information about dress codes, parking, personal use of the telephone, office hours, days off, and after-hours responsibilities.

Clarify exactly when the learner will be in the office and any deviations from the schedule. Establish the process and responsibility for notifying the office if the learner cannot attend scheduled sessions due to illness or other reasons. Determine how you can easily notify the learner if you are unexpectedly unavailable. Obtain a reliable phone number of the institutional contact person in case other problems arise. Such problems might include failure of the learner to arrive when expected, a sudden change in the office schedule, or not having the necessary evaluation forms.

Several days in advance of the learner's arrival, remind your office staff and partners of the start date. Distribute a copy of the learner's application or personal information and schedule. If you haven't already done so, brief the office staff on the learner's participation and duties, including learning experiences that may involve them and their areas of responsibility. Review with the receptionist how they will inform patients about the learner in the office and their role in patient care. Listen to the receptionist practice the presentation to make sure it is offered in a positive and affirmative fashion. Experience has shown that this initial introduction can "make or break" the experience. If your teaching plan includes the learner seeing same-day "work-in" patients, coach the receptionist or nurse making these appointments to deliver the message in a way that supports your teaching effort.

Determine where the learner will park and locate a space in the office for the learner to work and study. Equip the space as necessary with references, note pads, writing utensils, and access to telephone and computer. It is not expected that a learner will have their own telephone and computer, but they should have reliable accessibility. You may wish to gather all of the office forms that the learner will use in one place, and you or one of your staff should describe when and how to use them. Review with the staff what their roles will be in the learner's orientation. A picture sheet with photos, names, roles and locations may be useful for orienting learners to the office. Similarly, a picture and short biography about the learner may help staff and patients.

Block out time on your schedule for a learner orientation. On that day, have the learner arrive early or have him or her come the day before. Experience has shown that a minimum of 30 minutes is necessary for a meaningful orientation. Take time to write down what you will cover. Save this to use with other learners and add to it as experience with different learners identifies other orientation needs. Some preceptors ask previous learners to generate a listing of "things I wish I knew on day 1" as a means of helping future learners orient and accommodate more easily into their clinical setting.

Finally, to be efficient and maximize your enjoyment, identify at least two examination rooms, one each for yourself and the learner. This will enable the two of you to see different patients simultaneously. Before the learner arrives, make the decision about whether he or she will write or dictate their chart notes or use the electronic health record (if this is an option in your office). If you wish the learner to dictate, be prepared to give instruction on how the dictation system works and how you would like it done. Consider creating a de-identified template or example note for learners. Write the instructions down and save them in your orientation file for future use.

### ❖ When the Learner Arrives

*Learning About Each Other*
The first meeting with a new student or resident should address mutual expectations (3,4). As noted above, you should allow approximately 30 minutes on the first day to greet the learner and share information. Begin by telling the learner about yourself and your practice, why you chose your specialty, and the rewards it has given you. You may want to also describe why you are interested in having a learner in your office. Then ask some questions about the learner, such as where he or she is from, his or her reasons for entering medicine, and his or her career goals and if there are any particular goals associated with choosing this experience (see When the Learner Arrives Orientation Checklist in Appendix B on page 150).

*Previous Experiences*
Next, discuss the learner's previous rotations, clerkships, ambulatory experiences, and patient care responsibilities. The Clinical Skills Inventory in Appendix A on page 124 is a simple list of previous learning experiences completed by the learner before beginning the office-based experience. This tool quickly outlines learning needs and can be used to plan the educational content of the experience.

*Expectations and Achievement of Learning Goals*
This is a good time to review the institution's expectations with the learner as well as his or her own goals for the experience. One strategy to accomplish both tasks is to develop a learner contract (see Learner Contract in Appendex A on page 126). A learner contract outlines the learner's and your expectations for the experience and serves as a guide for your final evaluation of the learner. More simply, a learner contract is a statement of intent or purpose that is described in observable and measurable terms. Examples include the following:
- Performance expected of the learner, preceptor, or both
- Desired teaching strategies

- Realistic criteria for successful completion of the learning goals (what, where, when, and how)

*Consequences of Achieving or Not Achieving Learning Goals*
The learner should complete the learner contract as early as possible, preferably on the first day. After reviewing the learner's goals, you can modify the contract based on your judgment and previous experience. Specific strategies to address the content in the contract can be included. The contract is then reviewed and signed by you and the learner.

*Responsibilities*
Be as explicit as possible about the entire spectrum of responsibilities. Consider such mundane but important aspects as how to dress, where to park, through what doorway to enter the building, and where to store personal possessions, as well as expectations about writing or dictating notes, using the electronic health record, ordering tests and consultations, and following up with patients. You can save time if these general rules are written down for the learner and reviewed at the beginning of the experience. Remember to save all orientation materials in a file for subsequent learners. Additionally, be very explicit on the amount of time the student is "allocated" to see each patient.

*Scheduling*
Review the flow of patients through the office and how teaching will occur. For example, beginning students might be asked simply to observe initially, then be allowed to see selected patients on their own, reporting back after a specified time when you and the learner together can see each patient again. Residents may have a schedule of their "own" patients, or other arrangements can be made. For detailed information about scheduling and an example of an effective schedule, see Patient Scheduling, below.

*Teaching*
You may wish to tell the learner you will "teach on the fly" primarily by asking questions, role modeling, and directing the learner to the literature to

answer important content questions. Whatever approach is used, briefly describe what will occur and what the learner must do to make the process work. Models of different case-based–learning techniques are presented later in this book (see Chapter 5) and include the information needed to accomplish this task.

### Evaluation and Feedback

The learner needs to know about evaluation and feedback, including when and how it will occur and a clear idea of what criteria will be used for evaluation. Use this time to reassure the learner that informal feedback will be offered frequently during the experience, so the results of the final evaluation will not be unexpected. It is often a good idea to set aside time at this point for a mid-rotation feedback appointment. This commits you to providing the feedback and gives the learner specific information on how and when it will take place (see Chapter 8, Learner Feedback and Evaluation).

### Office Flow

You or your office manager should take a few minutes to provide an orientation to the office. Introduce the learner to all members of the office staff and provide an explanation of their duties and responsibilities. You might consider conducting your introductions in a way that simulates the flow of patients through the office, beginning with the receptionist, medical-record personnel, health aides, nurses, checkout staff, and others.

### Workspace and Notes

Define, if you can, the learner's workspace, including where they can sit, place their personal belongings, and perform charting. Review your expectations about charting or dictation and telephone, electronic health record and computer use. Show how they can access information, including textbooks, journals, and online materials.

*Examination Rooms*

Review the contents of a typical examination room, including the locations of gloves, gowns, stool cards, and examination instruments. If you expect the learner to fill out laboratory or radiology request forms, show the learner where they are located and how to fill them out. Other innovative ways to introduce the learner to an office is to have him or her actually "check in" as a patient. Using this technique, he or she meets the receptionist, fills out medical forms, is ushered into an examination room, is escorted to the laboratory, is given checkout materials, is taken to the checkout window, and is then sent to the laboratory or to the radiology department. There is no educational experience quite like being a patient.

*Informing Patients*

At the time the learner arrives, post notices for patients about the learner's participation around the reception area and at the front desk (see Patient Notice for Students in the Office and Patient Notice for Residents in the Office in Appendix A on pages 128-9). Many practices take photographs of their current learners and place them in the waiting area with the learner's name and title (i.e., student or resident physician). Create a short biography of the learners and offer it to patients when they arrive. Patients appreciate this type of personal knowledge about new faces in the office (see Biography of a Resident Physician in Appendix A on page 130). Ask the reception staff to tell patients that you are teaching a student or resident.

## ❖ Patient Scheduling

Proper patient scheduling for you and the learner can improve office and teaching efficiency. One example of efficient scheduling is the wave schedule (see The Wave Schedule in Table 3-1 and in Appendix B on page 152). This model begins with your usual schedule, but every second or third patient is asked to come to the office one appointment slot earlier, allowing you and the learner to see patients simultaneously. Patients need to be informed that their visit will be a "double visit" because they may have other appointments or meetings scheduled. After the visits are completed, your patient is discharged from the office and then you and the learner examine the second (learner's) patient together during the freed appointment slot. A typical schedule changed to a wave schedule might look like the one in Table 3-1.

This model allows physicians to see the same number of patients with a learner present, without necessarily extending the day. The wave schedule can be more intense for advanced learners (who can see every other patient) or less intense for novices (who need more time to write notes or read about patients during the day). The training program should provide you with guidelines as to the number of new and return patients the learner is expected to see. Be prepared to modify this when you have ascertained the learner's competency and efficiency. Obviously, this model requires the staff to call and ask selected patients to arrive early for their appointment or to inform patients when they are calling for an appointment. This is also an opportunity to explain that a learner is in the office, to inform patients of the possibility of an extended visit, and to obtain permission for the learner to see them.

## Table 3-1 Wave Schedule

| Time AM | Original Physician Schedule | Learner Wave Schedule | Physician Wave Schedule |
|---------|------------------------------|------------------------|--------------------------|
| 8:00–8:20 | Patient A | Patient A | Patient B |
| 8:20–8:40 | Patient B | Patient A | Patient A |
| 8:40–9:00 | Patient C | Writes note | Patient C |
| 9:00–9:20 | Patient D | Patient D | Patient E |
| 9:20–9:40 | Patient E | Patient D | Patient D |
| 9:40–10:00 | Patient F | Writes note | Patient F |
| 10:00–10:20 | Patient G | Patient G | Patient H |
| 10:20–10:40 | Patient H | Patient G | Patient G |
| 10:40–11:00 | Patient I | Writes note | Patient I |
| 11:00–11:20 | Patient J | Patient J | Patient K |
| 11:20–11:40 | Patient K | Patient J | Patient J |
| 11:40–Noon | Patient L | Writes note | Patient L |

Although this model demonstrates a schedule with appointments every 20 minutes, it is easily adaptable to schedules of any appointment length, provided that the slots are of equal length. In any case, review the schedule with learners at the beginning of each session. Point out who they will see, "prime" them with your expectations for the visit, and "frame" the visit by emphasizing the time limits and your expectations about what parts of the physical examination to perform and how the case is to be presented (see Strategies for Organizing the Office Visit in Chapter 4 on page 45 for for information about priming, framing, and patient-presentation format).

Obviously, the Wave schedule only works if you have a minimum of two examination rooms available to you; one for you and one for the learner. What can you do if you only have one examination room? Think of ways to activate the learner to avoid learner passivity and boredom (1). Activation may take many forms, including:

- Priming the learner to watch you perform a particular part of the examination (see Active Observation in Chapter 6 on page 79)
- Have the learner look up medications, dosages, and side effects as you are talking with the patient
- Have the learner begin to formulate a clinical question that will be the basis for an evidence-based medicine search (see Just in Time Learning in Chapter 6 on page 82)
- Have the learner review the patient note for trends in patient specific data such as blood pressure, weight, and hemoglobin $A_1c$ levels
- Ask the learner to measure vital signs or perform a particular part of the examination while you write prescriptions or the note (see Collaborative Examinations in Chapter 6 on page 78)

These are techniques that work best with very early or clinically inexperienced learners and for the most part are not suitable for more experienced students or residents. These learners need the opportunity to see patients independently, at least initially, to practice medicine under your supervision.

When arranging the learner's schedule, keep in mind his or her level of expertise and previous experiences. If possible, select patients who match the learner's abilities. Inexperienced learners do best seeing patients with a single, simple problem or patients with classical or typical presentations of common diseases. Select patients who are good historians, are "patient" patients, and who do not have major psychosocial issues. Complex patients can easily overwhelm novice learners. On the other hand, advanced learners like to be challenged with undifferentiated clinical problems, enabling them to practice in an environment that typifies clinical practice. Patients with multiple, complex medical problems are appropriate for these learners.

Another efficient scheduling model is the "work-in schedule." In this model, the learner is assigned to see a sufficient number of urgent work-in patients to meet the curricular goals of the experience. Alternatively, you can see the work-in patients and the learner can see some of the regularly scheduled patients if this arrangement better meets with the institution's expectations or with the learner contract.

## ❖ Ancillary Teaching Opportunities

Keep in mind that there may be other valuable learning experiences for the student, including the following:

- Home visits
- Hospice visits
- Nursing home visits
- Physical therapy visits
- Laboratory/blood drawing experience
- Giving injections (great experience during flu season)
- Patient-education encounters
- Working with the receptionist
- Working with the business manager
- Attending office business meetings
- Triaging patient telephone calls
- Chart audits for quality improvement

Although these experiences are not intended to replace the clinical experience in the office, they are often greatly appreciated by the learner as supplemental experiences. It will be more meaningful to the learner if you articulate the rationale for the experience and briefly review the experience afterward by asking the learner what they learned.

## ❖ When the Patients Arrive

Have the receptionist inform incoming patients that you are working with a learner today. Some offices prepare an inexpensive brochure or "newsletter" that describes the teaching program and introduces the learner to the patient (see Biography of a Resident Physician in Appendix A on page 130). Patients appreciate these informational pieces, particularly when they emphasize personal information about the learner. Some institutions will provide these for you and include a photograph of the learner. The receptionist should be prepared to answer any patient questions about the program and the learner in a positive and supportive fashion (see When the Patients Arrive Checklist in Appendix B on page 153).

Personally inform your patients that you are providing a learning experience in your office for a medical student or resident. Ask the patient's permission before bringing the learner into the examining room or before allowing the learner to see the patient independently. You may wish to ask permission to have the learner present the case findings to you in front of the patient. As discussed later, this technique can save you considerable teaching time and is typically appreciated by the patient (5,6) (see Presenting in the Room in Chapter 6 on page 76).

When introducing the learner, use positive language: "I have a medical student/resident physician working with me today. If it's OK with you, I'd like him/her to talk to you and examine you first. I will come in and see you afterwards." Most patients will react positively, particularly when it is presented by you in an affirmative fashion, and will be comfortable and willing to have the learner in the room. However, never assume this to be the case. Allow each patient to make the final determination.

If you teach frequently, consider informing new patients that you often work with learners. This sets the expectation for the office, even if the individual learners change over time.

Have the office staff inform you about any positive or negative feedback from the patients about the learner. Use this information in your feedback sessions with the learner. Nothing is as powerful as patient feedback to change learner behavior (7).

## ❖ After the Patients Leave

Whether you are teaching or not, you must appropriately document the patient's visit (and your involvement) in order to be eligible for reimbursement by Medicare (and other insurance carriers). Lack of proper documentation can lead to charges of Medicare fraud.

### Documentation Requirements for a Resident

Current Medicare rules permit a teaching physician (preceptor) to substantiate a bill based on the combination of the resident's and the teaching physician's documentation of a specific service. The teaching physician must clearly convey that he or she saw the patient and participated personally in the patient's care up to the level of the evaluation and management services billed. The teaching physician can confirm that he or she verified the findings in the resident's note and agree with findings as documented by the resident. The teaching physician can also indicate that he or she agrees with the diagnosis and plan as written by the resident. These rules permit a certain amount of time saved by using the resident's documentation as part of your own note. This will somewhat decrease the overall work associated with teaching by allowing you to receive some "service" for your educational endeavors. See Box 3-1 for an example of documentation.

### Documentation Requirements for a Student

The only documentation by medical students that may be used by the teaching physician is the review of systems (ROS) and past, family, and social histories (PFSH). Currently, the teaching physician may not refer to a medical student's documentation of physical examination findings or medical decision making in his or her note (8). These restrictions obviously will have an effect on office efficiency, but you can still use the student's note as a guide when dictating or writing your own note. Experienced preceptors frequently use the student's note in this way to be more efficient. One meticulously performed study documented a saving of 3.3 minutes of charting time per patient using this technique (9). Additionally, certain other strategies can be used to maximize efficiency in spite of these regulatory requirements (see the Wave Schedule in Table 3-1, and also see Presenting in the Room and Collaborative Examinations in Chapter 6 on pages 76 and 78 for other methods to help manage documentation requirements when a student is present).

---

### Box 3-1. Example of a Note by Attending Physician Dr. Smith Who Is Supervising Resident Physician Dr. Fox

I saw Mrs. Jones with Dr. Fox for dizziness associated with standing up quickly. She was recently started on hydrochlorothiazide for hypertension and has no history of blood or fluid loss. She is orthostatic as noted. Her cardiovascular and neurological examinations are normal. I agree that her symptoms are due to hydrochlorothiazide and that a chemistry panel and hematocrit should be done. See Dr. Fox's note as signed by me for more details. [Signed] Dr. Smith.

---

## REFERENCES

1. **DeWitt DE.** Incorporating medical students into your practice. Aust Fam Physician. 2006;35:24-6.
2. **Jain S.** Orienting family medicine residents and medical students to office practice. Fam Med. 2005;37:461-3.
3. **Skeff KM.** Enhancing teaching effectiveness and vitality in the ambulatory setting. J Gen Intern Med. 1988;3:S26-33.
4. **Lesky LG, Hershman WY.** Practical approaches to a major educational challenge. Training students in the ambulatory setting. Arch Intern Med. 1998;155:897-904.

5. **Anderson RJ, Cyran E, Schilling L, et al.** Outpatient case presentations in the conference room versus examination room: results from two randomized controlled trials. Am J Med. 2002;113:657-62.
6. **Rogers HD, Carline JD, Paauw DS.** Examination room presentations in general internal medicine clinic: patients' and students' perceptions. Acad Med. 2003;78:945-9.
7. **Cope DW, Linn LS, Leake BD, Barrett PA.** Modification of residents' behavior by preceptor feedback of patient satisfaction. J Gen Intern Med. 1986;1:394-8.
8. **Chappelle KG, Blanchard SH, Ramirez-Williams MF, Fields SA.** Medical students and Health Care Financing Administration documentation guidelines. Fam Med. 2000; 32:459-61.
9. **Usatine RP, Tremoulet PT, Irby D.** Time-efficient preceptors in ambulatory care settings. Acad Med. 2000;75:639-42.

# 4

# Teaching Skills and Organizational Techniques for Office-Based Teaching

T his chapter begins with a description of meaningful patient responsibility and an overview of the personal characteristics of outstanding clinical teachers. This is followed by descriptions of useful pre-visit organizational strategies. (See Summary of the Learning Experience in Appendix B on page 154 for an outline of this chapter and Chapters 5 and 6.)

## ❖ Meaningful Responsibility

To create a truly effective learning experience, students and residents need meaningful responsibility. The amount of responsibility depends on the learner's level of training and your best judgment. Nevertheless, most learners need the opportunity to see patients independently, collect data, make preliminary decisions, and then report back to you. As the preceptor, you need to balance between having learners "see it all" (with you) and having them work on their own with fewer patients. Although there is educational merit in having learners watch you interact with patients, entirely observational experiences lead to frustration and boredom (1). Of course, there is a natural tendency to want learners to be under your direct observation. Most clinical teachers are concerned about patient satisfaction, want to provide care personally, and want to stay on schedule. Learners do benefit from this experience, termed "legitimate peripheral participation," and many trades include this form of education as part of apprenticeship training. However, combining this approach with ones that allow the learners increasingly independent supervised responsibility increases their learning. As previously noted, patient satisfaction with learners is usually high; by using the techniques presented in this text, you can personalize your care and minimize delays in your schedule.

## ❖ Characteristics of Effective Clinical Teachers

Good teaching makes a difference. Students exposed to good teachers have better overall performance on the clerkship and score higher on end of clerkship examinations and on Step 2 of the United States Medical Licensing Examination (2-4). Good teachers can positively influence career choices just as poor teachers can negatively influence career decisions (5). While this means that there are plenty of good reasons to be a good teacher, few of us are naturally good teachers and most of us need help in developing our teaching skills. Fortunately, we now know the attributes that are associated with effective teaching and most of them are simple, straight forward strategies that can be mastered with practice.

One source of information on effective teaching comes from surveys of graduating medical students and residents. National teaching experts and direct observation of experienced teachers have confirmed the validity of the survey results (6-11). Excellent ambulatory teachers were described as those physicians who are good at the following actions:

- Communicating expectations
- Selecting appropriate patients
- Stimulating interest enthusiastically
- Interacting skillfully with patients
- Role modeling desired behaviors
- Involving the learner in the teaching process

- Limiting the number of teaching points
- Giving feedback

Other characteristics associated with teaching effectiveness are providing opportunities to learn and practice clinical skills, opportunities to observe the preceptor practice ethical medicine, and ones to practice evidence-based medicine (12).

*Communicating Expectations*

Clearly communicating your expectations is best done during the office orientation. Be as explicit as possible, and organize your orientation by using a checklist (see When the Learner Arrives Orientation Checklist in Appendix B on page 150). You might involve your office members in the orientation process. You can improve your future effectiveness by asking the learner at the end of the rotation if there was anything else about teaching and expectations that would have been useful in the orientation.

*Stimulating Interest Enthusiastically*

Stimulating learner interest is a vital component of establishing a positive learning environment (10). Allow your natural enthusiasm for patient care to be expressed through your words and actions. Unusual aspects of problems should be shared with the learner; compare past experiences and invite learners to share their reactions (a technique known as reflection) to issues. For the novice learner, all patients present special challenges and even repetitive patient problems can be stimulating if different aspects of care are highlighted in the discussion. For example, one patient with diabetes can be the springboard for a discussion on natural history, a second could elicit a lesson on prevention, and a third may illustrate compliance issues. Through your actions, the learner will see each patient as being unique and presenting a different opportunity to learn more about medicine. As noted by a respected educator, "We suspect that the best teachers do not necessarily impart more factual knowledge (facts which may be obsolete in a few years), but rather they engender a learning climate that makes learning fun, enjoyable and exciting" (3).

*Interacting Skillfully with Patients*

Excellent clinical teachers are knowledgeable and clinically competent, have good rapport with patients, and are perceived as excellent role models (13). You can provide a valuable educational experience to learners by demonstrating a mastery of the traits you acquired through years of experience (14). Occasionally, take advantage of this wealth of talent by having the learner observe you interacting with patients. First, "set the stage" by telling the learner what to look for and why it is important, and afterward provide an opportunity for the learner to describe what took place (15). Then observe the learner as he or she takes the opportunity to practice the skill that you have demonstrated and provide feedback (see Active Observation in Chapter 6 on page 79). For example, before counseling a patient about smoking cessation, ask the learner to observe you, with the expectation that he or she will counsel the next patient who needs similar information. You will watch the learner's counseling efforts and later provide him or her with a specific evaluation of the performance.

*Involving the Learner*

Active observation, as described above, is one method of involving the learner. Ask the learner to identify his or her knowledge and skill limitations and help them organize experiences to address these deficiencies (7). Give learners assignments that address their learning needs and ask them to report back with the results of their research (see Self-Directed [Independent] Learning in Chapter 6 on page 82).

One useful teaching strategy is the educational prescription (see Educational Prescription Form in Appendix A on page 131). When a learning issue becomes apparent, you can take a prescription pad and write out the problem or the assignment. For example, "Is a seven-day course of antibiotics superior to a three-day course for an uncomplicated UTI?" or "Read about the treatment of uncomplicated cystitis." The prescription also should denote a time frame for completing the assignment and how it should be completed, e.g., "Provide a five-minute summary of the evidence tomorrow morning" or "Make a five-minute presentation on cystitis by the end of the day." The use of a formalized prescription clarifies and documents expectations. For example, you may ask a student to "read more about the risk factors" of the disease process just encountered in the office. The preceptor assumes that this is a clear instruction and that the learner will be ready to discuss the topic the next day, but we have sometimes found that the learner hears this instruction as an invitation that they can decline.

You can model key attitudes of active inquiry and lifelong learning by demonstrating patient-centered clinical problem solving. This can be done by verbally framing (with the learner) the clinical question that needs to be answered, for example, "Is finasteride more effective than doxazosin in the treatment of benign prostatic hypertrophy?" Then demonstrate how the question can be answered by using data from the medical literature or other sources of reliable information.

## *Limiting the Number of Teaching Points*

Limiting the number of teaching points is an effetive strategy used by a number of experienced teachers (16). In the enthusiam to teach, the temptation is to share everything you know, but this can easily overwhelm the learner. Instead, focus on a few main points; experience has shown that this often leds to greater learning. The teaching points, or "take-home messages," should be general rules that can apply to other situations. Using this strategy produces learning that is more memorable and more easily transferable to new situations

## *Role Modeling Desired Behaviors*

Role modeling is an integral component of medical education and an important factor in shaping the values, attitudes, behavior, and ethics of learners. Indeed 90% of students identify one or more role models during medical school, almost all during the clinical years (17). In a study of teaching physicians who were identified as excellent role models by internal medicine residents, several characteristics were identified that distinguished them from physicians who were not chosen as role models. Excellent role models were more likely to stress the importance of the doctor-patient relationship, to spend more time on the psychosocial aspects of medicine, and to give more in-depth and specific feedback to learners (18). Excellent role models also were more likely to engage in activities that built relationships with residents (e.g., asking about career plans, family, and outside interests and providing personal information about their lives). Characteristics that were not associated with being an excellent role model included age, sex, academic rank, additional education beyond the medical degree, and part-time/full-time status. Interestingly, a strong knowledge base was a less important determinant of being an excellent role model than were traits such as the ability to promote understanding, and personality traits such as patience and being "nonthreatening" (17).

This information suggests that all community-based physicians can be excellent role models. The task of being a role model can be made easier by remembering that learners in your office are actually trying on your job and lifestyle "for size." Be an effective advocate for your specialty by demonstrating enthusiasm for what you are doing. Keep in mind that students and residents learn best from watching experts deal with difficult situations. Allow this to happen by inviting the learner in the room when you anticipate such a situation. Afterward, discuss the encounter with the learner to maximize the discovery process. Learners appreciate the opportunity to see an experienced physician working within a long-term physician-patient relationship. For many, this will be their first experience in the office setting, and an opportunity to observe your interaction with an established patient will be both educational and motivational.

Comments from students and residents shed further light on good teaching. As expected, effective ambulatory teachers possess a "broad knowledge of medicine," but also good teachers are "good people." As a group, effective teachers enjoy teaching and patient care, demonstrate concern for their patients, are personal and approachable, show respect for others, and are enthusiastic (10).

### ❖ Selecting Appropriate Patients

Selecting patients to participate in office-based teaching requires both thoughtful reflection and compromise. Expert teachers try to select patients for students that maximize teaching and learning but also maintain practice flow and efficiency and the relationship between preceptor and patient. With this in mind, experienced preceptors often steer students away from "difficult patients" that are less likely to be satisfied with their visit even in the absence of learners (19). More appropriate patients for novice learners are those who are good historians and who do not have major psychosocial issues. On the other hand, advanced learners like to be challenged, enabling them to practice in an environment that typifies clinical practice. Patients with multiple, complex medical problems are appropriate for these learners.

## ❖ Strategies for Organizing the Office Visit

Learners in general, and students in particular, often have trouble deciding how to organize the process of collecting and then presenting patient data. Compared with the hospital environment in which time is not a factor, the ambulatory setting presents unique challenges of addressing patient concerns and collecting information in a limited amount of time. The following paragraphs describe tools and tips that can help organize the learner's visit with the patient (see Instructions to Help the Learner Organize the Patient Visit in Appendix A on page 132).

### Data Collection and Patient Presentation

One of us (LEP) has created the organizational scheme in Box 4-1 for learners at the University of Washington. To be used effectively, you should take a few minutes to go over this organizational framework with the learner, possibly during the orientation. To help the learner, this framework is formatted as a series of tables that can be copied and written on to guide the data collection (see Tools to Help the Learner Organize the Patient Visit in Appendix A on page 135). For learners having trouble making a patient presentation, the Patient Presentation Format for Learners in Appendix A on page 137 also can be used as a guide. The time spent in acclimating the student to the organizational framework and presentation format will be repaid in increased efficiency during the course of the rotation.

**Box 4-1. Data Collection Scheme for Learners**

**What?**

▶ Elicit the patient's agenda: "What should we talk about today?"

**Why?**

▶ Elicit the patient's attribution or understanding of the problem: "What do you think is causing this? What do you think should be done?"

**Why?**

▶ Identify the most likely hypothesis and supporting data. Be able to answer the question, "What is the supporting evidence?"

**What else?**

▶ Create a prioritized and weighted differential diagnosis. Again, be able to answer the question, "What is the supporting evidence?"

**What now?**

▶ Determine the immediate next steps: "What history, parts of the focused examination, and tests need to be done? What are the treatment options? What patient education needs to be done?"

Developing a related strategy, Peltier and colleagues at Dartmouth developed and evaluated the use of Focus Scripts for medical students (20). Similar to the organizational scheme used at the University of Washington, scripts are frameworks to help organize complex knowledge into simpler patterns. Focus Scripts address the difficulty students have in assembling relevant information in the short time frame of the outpatient visit. They are paper-based guides specifically designed for the early clinical student beginning an office experience to help the learner concentrate on the specific task of doing a focused history and physical examination. A generic acute and chronic problem script and examples of disease specific scripts for common acute and chronic conditions were provided to the learners (See Appendix A, Tools for Preceptors on pages 139-40). Students who used the scripts were more likely to perform and record appropriate history and physical examinations findings, have greater clarity of diagnosis, and incorporate appropriate laboratory data.

*Priming*

Another organizational strategy that can be used to focus the visit is "priming." Priming involves providing the learner with pertinent patient-specific background information just before seeing the patient and directing the student to perform specific tasks of patient care (21). For example, if a learner is about to see a patient with chest pain, you might briefly (for 1–2 minutes) review with the learner the most common causes of chest pain and aspects of the history and physical examination that would be helpful in differentiating between causes. Remember that asking the learner is better than "telling" because you learn about their level of function while priming them (e.g., "What are the causes of chest pain you should consider in a 35-year-old athletic woman?"). For patients with chronic medical problems, priming might involve reviewing health maintenance or disease screening needs just before the visit. Priming can be used when seeing complex patients with multiple medical problems by having the learner review what might be the most important outcome of the office visit (see Box 4-2).

---

### Box 4-2. How a Learner May Be Primed for a Visit

▶ Mrs. Jones is a healthy 28-year-old woman and is here for her yearly examination. At her age, what are the important screening issues to be covered?

▶ Mr. Smith is a 50-year-old man with chronic lung disease and is here after a brief hospitalization for pneumonia. What symptoms should we look for today, and what parts of the physical examination should we focus on?

▶ Miss Doe is a 60-year-old woman with hypertension treated with hydrochlorothiazide and is here with the complaint of dizziness. In her age group, what are the important considerations in the differential diagnosis? What inquires should we make about her medication?

> **Box 4-3. Priming**
>
> ▶ Giving the learner critical information to help initiate the visit.

A brief discussion before the visit that includes the strategy of priming will avoid the learner performing a complete history and physical examination by focusing on the appropriate examination for the problem at hand in the allotted time (see Box 4-3).

> **Box 4-4. Framing**
>
> ▶ Setting expectations and time limits for what you want the learner to accomplish during his or her time with the patient.

*Framing*

Another organizational strategy that increases the efficiency of the learner is "framing." Framing is setting parameters for the visit such that the learner will accomplish a focused task. For example, learners can be given specific instructions on what to accomplish during the visit: "I want you to take a history of the patient's chest pain, do a focused examination, and report back to me in 15 minutes."

You will find that not all learners need to be "primed" or have the visit "framed," but most medical students and beginning residents will benefit from this approach (see Box 4-4).

REFERENCES

1. **Krajic Kachur E.** Observation during early clinical exposure - an effective instructional tool or a bore? Med Educ. 2003;37:88-9.
2. **Stern DT, Williams BC, Gill A, et al.** Is there a relationship between attending physicians' and residents' teaching skills and students' examination scores? Acad Med. 2000;75:1144-6.

3. **Griffith CH 3rd, Georgesen JC, Wilson JF.** Six-year documentation of the association between excellent clinical teaching and improved students' examination performances. Acad Med. 2000;75:S62-4

4. **Roop SA, Pangaro L.** Effect of clinical teaching on student performance during a medicine clerkship. Am J Med. 2001;110:205-9.

5. **Griffith CH 3rd, Georgesen JC, Wilson JF.** Specialty choices of students who actually have choices: the influence of excellent clinical teachers. Acad Med. 2000;75:278-82.

6. **Wilkerson L, Armstrong E, Lesky L.** Faculty development for ambulatory teaching. J Gen Intern Med. 1990;5(Suppl):S44-53.

7. **Skeff KM.** Enhancing teaching effectiveness and vitality in the ambulatory setting. J Gen Intern Med. 1988;3(Suppl):S26-33.

8. **Roberts KB.** Educational principles of community-based education. Pediatrics. 1996;98:1259-63.

9. **Gjerde CL, Coble RJ.** Resident and faculty perceptions of effective clinical teaching in family practice. J Fam Prac. 1982;14:323-7.

10. **Irby DM, Ramsey PG, Gillmore GM, Schaad D.** Characteristics of effective clinical teachers of ambulatory care medicine. Acad Med. 1991;66:54-5.

11. **Whitman N, Magill MK.** Is attending a teaching skills workshop worth your time? Fam Med. 1998;30:255-6.

12. **Elnicki DM, Kolarik R, Bardella I.** Third-year medical students' perceptions of effective teaching behaviors in a multidisciplinary ambulatory clerkship. Acad Med. 2003;78:815-9.

13. **Irby DM.** Teaching and learning in ambulatory care settings: a thematic review of the literature. Acad Med. 1995;70:898-931.

14. **Loftus TH, McLeod PJ, Snell LS.** Faculty perceptions of effective ambulatory care teaching. J Gen Intern Med. 1993;8:575-7.

15. **Epstein RM, Cole DR, Gawinski BA, et al.** How students learn from community-based preceptors. Arch Fam Med. 1998;7:149-54.

16. **Heidenreich C, Lye P, Simpson D, Lourich M.** The search for effective and efficient ambulatory teaching methods through the literature. Pediatrics. 2000;105:231-7.

17. **Wright S, Wong A, Newill C.** The impact of role models on medical students. J Gen Intern Med. 1997;12:53-6.

18. **Wright SM, Kern DE, Kolodner K, et al.** Attributes of excellent attending physician role models. N Engl J Med. 1998;339:1986-93.

19. **Simon SR, Davis D, Peters AS, et al.** How do precepting physicians select patients for teaching medical students in the ambulatory primary care setting? J Gen Intern Med. 2003;18:730-5.

20. **Peltier D, Regan-Smith M, Wofford J, et al.** Teaching focused histories and physical exams in ambulatory care: a multi-institutional randomized trial. Teach Learn Med. 2007;19:244-50.

21. **McGee SR, Irby DM.** Teaching in the outpatient clinic: practical tips. J Gen Intern Med. 1997;12(Suppl):S34-40.

# 5

# Case-Based Learning

This chapter first answers the questions, "What is case-based learning?" and "How can I teach in the office in a way that supports the learner?" Then it reviews seven precepting models:

- The Microskills Model
- The "Aunt Minnie" Model
- Modeling Problem Solving
- The One-Minute Observation
- Learner-Centered Precepting
- SNAPPS Model of Learner-Centered Precepting
- Reflection

Also see Chapter 6 for models on how to make more efficient use of the available time.

## ❖ What Is Case-Based Learning?

The traditional model of case-based learning is familiar to most physicians. A learner presents a case to you after independently gathering the patient data. You then must create educational opportunities for the learner that relate to the case and provide care for the patient. These tasks might be accomplished by doing the following:

- Role modeling ("Watch me care for the patient")
- Questioning ("Tell me what you think and why")
- Performing expert consultation ("Ask me what you need to know")
- Mini-lecturing ("I will tell you what I know about this topic")
- Modeling problem solving ("I will think out loud about this case")
- Encouraging self-directed, independent learning ("What do you need to read about to understand this case?")
- Assigning teacher-directed, independent learning ("I think you should look this up")

Most preceptors use a combination of techniques, and with experience preceptors learn to choose which model is right for a specific situation.

## ❖ The Microskills Model (One-Minute Preceptor)

Neher and coworkers (1) have broken down case-based precepting into five microskills that facilitate learning (see Summary of the Microskills Model for Preception in Appendix B on page 156). This method uses the technique of questioning to understand and address learner and patient needs efficiently and effectively. It allows you 1) to assess what the learner does and does not know, 2) to instruct the learner, and 3) to provide feedback more efficiently.

The Microskills can be used with nearly any level of learner skill. The five rules are listed in Box 5-1.

---

### Box 5-1. The Microskills Model

**1. Get a commitment**
- ▶ "What do you think is going on with this patient?"

**2. Probe for supporting evidence**
- ▶ "Why do you think that?"

*continued*

3. **Teach general rules**
   ▶ "Always do this when you see a similar case"
4. **Reinforce what was done right**
   ▶ "Here is what you did right, and this is why it is important"
5. **Correct mistakes**
   ▶ "I will tell you what you can do better"
   ▶ "I will tell you how to do it better"

*Get a Commitment*

The first microskill asks the learner to commit to some decision or plan of action. The cue to use this microskill is when the learner pauses after presenting a patient, waiting for you to offer an explanation of the findings or a course of action. At this point, instead of taking over the case and solving the problem and inadvertently missing a teaching opportunity, you should ask, "What do you think is going on?" Other appropriate questions might include, "What do you want to do" or "How would you manage this?" Asking for a commitment encourages the learner to feel more responsible for the patient, forces active learning, and engenders a sense of collaboration with you. Learners who make mistakes reveal gaps in their knowledge or judgment that can be addressed by you, either with a short explanation or with a follow-up reading assignment. See Box 5-2 for helpful and unhelpful examples of approaches to obtaining committments.

**Box 5-2. Helpful Approaches to Getting a Commitment**
   ▶ "What do you think is going on with this patient?"
   ▶ "Why do you think the patient continues to be hypertensive on three medications?"
   ▶ "What do you want to accomplish during this visit?"

*continued*

These questions are characterized by expecting the learner to offer an explanation, not just answering "yes" or "no"; he or she must elaborate his or her knowledge for you.

**Unhelpful Approaches to Getting a Commitment**

- ▶ "Sounds like pneumonia, don't you think?"
- ▶ "Did you consider CHF the cause of his dyspnea?"

These questions do not demand elaboration of knowledge by the learner; they can be answered "yes" or "no," and the answer is often prompted by the nature of the question.

*Probe for Supporting Evidence*

After you get the learner to make a commitment, ask the learner for the evidence that supports the commitment. Instead of saying, "You are right" or "You are wrong," ask questions like "What were the major findings that led you to that diagnosis?" or "Why did you choose furosemide rather than hydrochlorothiazide?" Questions help the learner reflect on the mental steps that were used to make the commitment. It is important to remember that probing for more information is not the same as "grilling" learners, and it helps to emphasize to the learner that this is a process to help them "think out loud." It also gives you a chance to analyze a learner's diagnostic abilities by understanding how the learner came to his or her conclusion. The core of this model is to first diagnose the learner. These first two steps are essential to doing this. They help you find out what the learner is thinking and help you avoid a situation where the learner is trying to guess what you want to hear. See Box 5-3 for helpful and unhelpful approaches to probing for evidence.

The skillful use of questions is an important technique used by experienced clinicians to teach and evaluate learners. Questions that allow for a small range of potentially correct answers are helpful for early learners. As the student's ability increases, the use of open-ended questions allows for broader ranges of potentially correct answers and a deeper probing of knowledge and judgment. Whitman and Schwenk (2) have described five

---

**Box 5-3.**

**Helpful Approaches to Probing for Supporting Evidence**

- ▶ "What about his presentation led you to this diagnosis?"
- ▶ "How did you decide that Mrs. Smith has pneumonia?"
- ▶ "What did you find on exam that makes you think this is a surgical abdomen?"
- ▶ "What were the factors that made you consider esophageal reflux rather than cardiac ischemia?"

These questions are characterized by asking the learner to demonstrate his or her thinking as it pertains to the case at hand. The learner must synthesize collected data and content knowledge to justify the diagnosis.

**Unhelpful Approaches to Probing for Supporting Evidence**

- ▶ "What are the possible causes of dyspnea on exertion?"
- ▶ "I don't think this is PID. Do you have any other ideas?"
- ▶ "This seems like a clear case of gout to me; how about you?"
- ▶ "What are the five most common bacterial causes of community-acquired pneumonia?"

These unhelpful questions are characterized by either having the learner create "lists" of diagnoses that may not be pertinent to the patient's problem or are "leading" questions that do not permit thoughtful consideration of the problem.

---

levels of questions useful in teaching and assessment; these are listed on page 146 with illustrative examples. Some of these categories of questions can be incorporated easily into the Microskills model. As highlighted by the box, the need to use certain types of questions may diagnose a poorly performed patient presentation, an ineffective orientation to the task, or both.

Questions coupled with immediate feedback are powerful teaching tools that, with practice, can be mastered by any preceptor. These questions also make excellent evaluation tools. When used sequentially, they allow you to assess the skill level of the learner, i.e., is the learner capable of only reporting the data or can he or she synthesize, justify, and demonstrate good judgment and decision-making skills? (See The RIME Evaluation Framework in Chapter 8 on page 112 for more information on this evaluation scheme.)

*Teach the General Rule*

Whenever possible, attempt to teach a general rule (3,4). General rules represent teaching scripts or "pearls" that are often presented effortlessly as they represent learning points gleaned from clinical experience. They commonly can be presented in one or two sentences. When something is offered as a general rule, it is more memorable and easily transferable to other cases than if offered as a patient-specific plan. Importantly, it is not imperative to "teach" something with each patient encounter. If the learner has done well, give positive feedback and save the formal teaching for another case. See Box 5-4 for helpful and unhelpful approaches to teaching general rules.

---

**Box 5-4.**

**Helpful Approaches to Teaching General Rules**

▶ "If a young adult has mechanical low-back pain, X-rays are usually not helpful."

▶ "It is helpful to address code status while patients are still healthy so that you can have a meaningful discussion."

▶ "When following up a case of pneumonia, remember that the infiltrates on the chest X-ray might not clear for 4 to 6 weeks. It is best to postpone the follow-up X-ray until after that time."

These questions are characterized by creating "rules of thumb" that can be applied reasonably to similar cases. They are short and to the point. The learner can be challenged to look up the scientific rationale for these rules as an independent learning assignment.

*continued*

**Unhelpful Approaches That Fail to Teach a General Rule**

▶ "Mr. Smith does not need a back X-ray today."

▶ "Why don't we discuss code status with Mrs. Jones today?"

▶ "Arrange for Mr. Doe to have his repeat chest X-ray at the end of the month."

▶ "I always treat pneumonia with two antibiotics because patients seem to do better."

▶ "I never give a flu and pneumonia vaccination at the same time. It might make the patient sick."

These examples address a specific problem and do not provide a general approach. They may also represent an unsupported, idiosyncratic approach to patient care. It often takes an insightful physician to recognize and correct this approach.

*Reinforce What Was Done Right*

This is sometimes referred to as "catching the learner doing something well." When the learner does well, reinforce what was done correctly by providing positive and specific feedback (see Feedback Tips in Chapter 8 on page 99). Even learners who are doing well may not recognize which elements of their behavior are helpful and thus which behaviors to continue. Positive feedback helps promote self-esteem and builds confidence and probably heightens awareness to corrective criticism when it is offered. Positive feedback should not be mistaken for general praise ("You did a good job with that last patient") but should be explicit, reinforcing desired behaviors. Effective positive feedback also includes a probable outcome of the observed behavior and provides a rationale for continuing it. For example, "You were very empathic with that patient, and she responded by providing important information in the history." See Box 5-5 for helpful and unhelpful approaches to reinforcing what the learner did right.

**Box 5-5.**

**Helpful Approaches to Reinforcing What Was Done Right**

► "You evaluated this in a stepwise fashion and considered the patient's preferences in your suggestions. As a result, she is likely to be compliant with our recommendations."

► "You did a good job noting the possible role of medication side effects in the diagnosis. This helped us avoid unnecessary tests."

These statements are characterized by providing specific praise that targets a specific action or behavior and the associated real or potential outcome of that action or behavior.

**Unhelpful Approaches That Do Not Reinforce What Was Done Right**

► "Strong work!"

► "You did a great job on that last case."

General praise that does not specify the precise action or behavior that was helpful (or how it was likely to be helpful) characterizes unhelpful feedback. The learner will not know exactly what was good, why it was good, or how to duplicate it.

*Correct Mistakes*

Learners make mistakes; when they do, supply corrective feedback. Remember that learners rarely make mistakes on purpose; most errors that persist are the result of insufficient feedback. For the feedback to be effective, you must choose an appropriate time and place to present the criticism to the learner. It is useful to begin by having learners review their own performance. Most learners have remarkable insight into their weaknesses and tend to be harder on themselves than their supervisors. Follow up the learner's comments with your own observations. Attempt to frame the observation of the mistake as "not the best" rather than "bad" or "wrong." Then provide specific guidance on improvement, e.g., by saying "You might be more successful next time this happens if you try..." and by giving them an opportunity to practice. See Box 5-6 for helpful and unhelpful approaches to correcting mistakes.

---

## Box 5-6.

### Helpful Approaches to Correcting Mistakes

▶ "I agree that Goodpasture's is a possible diagnosis but bacterial sinusitis is much more likely based on disease prevalence and lack of other findings. Next time, consider common conditions first."

▶ "Your diagnosis is correct, but she cannot afford the medication you recommended. Next time consider the patient's financial circumstances when recommending medications."

This feedback is characterized by identifying a specific behavior or action that needs correction and what needs to be done to improve the next time.

### Unhelpful Approaches to Correcting Mistakes

▶ "I can't believe you know so little for a fourth-year student."

▶ "You actually ordered that?"

These unhelpful statements are characterized as being vague or judgmental and are not accompanied with advice on how to improve. Avoid these kinds of statements. (See Chapter 8 for more information on giving feedback.)

---

*Why Should I Use the Microskills Model?*

What makes this model so appealing, to both preceptors and learners, is that it de-emphasizes the effect of transferring "new knowledge" and showcases everyday patient-management skills.

This precepting model can be easily learned in workshops lasting less than one hour and is modestly associated with improved student ratings of teaching skills (5). The Microskills model is a more efficient model of teaching, better facilitates your ability to make the correct diagnoses, and fosters greater confidence in rating student performance (6,7). The

Microskills model is associated with more teaching about the patient's specific illness including differential diagnosis, testing, and disease presentation (8). Preceptors who use the microskills have improved confidence in their feedback skills, and give more specific feedback to learners (7). Finally, preceptors trained in the Microskills model spent more time listening to the presentation and soliciting understanding of the learners' thinking and less time eliciting data from the learner (5). See Box 5-7 for a list of what you can accomplish by using the Microskills Model.

---

### Box 5-7. What Preceptors Can Accomplish with the Microskills Model

► Diagnosis of the patient by asking questions
► Analysis of the learner by getting a commitment and probing for evidence
► Instruction by providing general rules and feedback

The first two microskills listed on page 52 analyze learner knowledge and reasoning by asking for a commitment and by probing for supporting evidence. The last three microskills, listed on page 53, offer instruction that is individualized to meet the learner's needs (i.e., by teaching general rules, reinforcing what was done right, and correcting mistakes).

---

### ❖ The "Aunt Minnie" Model

Traditional case-based teaching, as described previously, involves three basic steps: the learner collects data from the patient; he or she reports the data to you, and, through a series of questions and answers, creates and prioritizes (with you) a differential diagnosis and plan. Cunningham and coworkers (11) have suggested an alternative, very quick model based on pattern recognition, otherwise known as the "Aunt Minnie" model (see Summary of the "Aunt Minnie Model of Precepting in Appendix B on page 157). "Aunt Minnie" is the name used by Sackett and coworkers (12) to describe a process of pattern recognition, i.e., if she dresses and walks like

Aunt Minnie, she probably is Aunt Minnie, even if you cannot see her face (12). This model is particularly effective when time is short and the case is straightforward. After the learner has collected the data from the patient, he or she is asked to present only the chief complaint and the most likely diagnosis. Typically, the learner will report the correct diagnosis and you can confirm this immediately. When the learner is wrong, brief and specific feedback is provided. This model works well with common conditions and allows you to expose the learner to more problems, increasing their depth of clinical experience.

With practice, the learner can quickly formulate the diagnosis and mentally summarize the data that support it (11). As learners and preceptors become more comfortable with this model, the nature of the teaching-learning dialog focuses on problem solving, rather than reporting a detailed history and physical examination, and more efficient teaching (13).

Some educators have expressed concerns that the student or resident will not learn how to do a complete history and physical examination and will be taught to make "snap judgments" rather than to consider carefully all aspects of the case. While premature closure can be an issue, the advice of Sackett and coworkers (12) is illuminating: "The student should be taught to do a complete history and physical examination, and then be taught to never use it." The skill of pattern recognition is a strategy used by experienced clinicians to evaluate common problems. If this teaching strategy is unsuccessful, you can always return to the beginning, ask the patients more questions, and demonstrate how to follow up new clues with an appropriate and focused physical examination. The learner then can see how detailed questioning and a directed examination fit properly into the scheme of caring for patients.

One of the benefits of the "Aunt Minnie" model is the provision of immediate, specific feedback to the learner, e.g., "You are right, the patient has acute otitis media" or "You were mistaken, the patient's tympanic membranes are normal, but the external ear canal is red and swollen; it's probably an external otitis. Go back and look again before the patient leaves the room." See Box 5-8 for a list of factors that facilitate the "Aunt Minnie" model's effectiveness.

With practice, the learner will be able to distinguish "Aunt Minnie" cases from those requiring a more detailed presentation and discussion.

---

**Box 5-8. Factors That Facilitate the "Aunt Minnie" Model's Effectiveness**

▶ The problem should be straightforward.

▶ The preceptor must see the patient.

▶ The preceptor must know the diagnosis; if the preceptor is uncertain about the diagnosis, he or she must be willing to admit it.

---

## ❖ Modeling Problem Solving

Another form of case-based learning is modeling problem solving; "thinking out loud" in front of the learner. This technique is particularly helpful when time is a factor or when the case is too complex for the learner (3,4). Examples include 1) reviewing diagnostic hunches and considering the pros and cons of each or 2) providing a rationale for a diagnostic or treatment decision. You can do this with the learner before entering the examination room or in front of the patient. Many patients report that they appreciate hearing their case discussed with learners because it adds to their own understanding (see Presenting in the Room in Chapter 6 on page 76).

This is a passive form of learning, but when framed correctly with the statement "I am going to think out loud for you" can be a valuable way to demonstrate how an expert clinician synthesizes data, prioritizes hunches, and plans the diagnostic and treatment components of care. In a sense, it is what you are asking the learner to do when using the Microskills. When you model problem solving, you can follow the Microskills model by making a vocal commitment and providing supporting data from the history and physical examination, and you might even have time to teach a general rule.

## ❖ The One-Minute Observation

This is a powerful, case-based, educational strategy proposed by Ferenchick and coworkers (14). It describes how to conduct a brief observation of a learner performing a specific clinical skill, such as collecting part of a history or performing part of the physical examination. Over time, and through the use of several "one-minute observations," much of the learner's history taking and physical examining can be observed (see Summary of the One-Minute Observation in Appendix B on page 158). This process allows you to observe, first hand, the learner's level of performance without the commitment of large blocks of time. The steps involved in successfully using this strategy are:

- Explain the purpose of the observation to the learner
- Explain how the observation will occur
- Select one skill for observation
- Inform the patient of your plan and purpose
- Observe for a brief period of time without interrupting
- Leave the room and have the learner join you when finished with the patient
- Provide immediate feedback
- Use the information gained about the learner to plan your teaching
- Repeat the process observing other skills

Observing the clinical skills of the learner means that feedback is based on first-hand data. Learners at all levels appreciate the opportunity to receive feedback, and this particular technique is well received by them. Some preceptors have created a checklist for the major parts of the history or physical examination they wish to observe first hand (see Feedback Note in Appendix A on page 141). Over time, each item on the list is observed and checked off (or a notation is made next to the item so that it can be referred to when providing feedback at a later time).

Closely related to the one-minute observation is the "mini-goals" model used by one of us (DED) and Doug Paauw at the University of Washington. In this model, you ask the learner to focus on a specific learning task for the day or week. For example, "Today let's work on history-taking skills. I'll watch you do just the history on one or two patients today and then give you feedback." You then watch the learner perform that task and provide specific instructive comments. At subsequent teaching sessions, the two of you may agree to work on different skills, such as the physical examination, patient education, or the visit "wrap-up." This technique tends to focus the precepting, to increase specific feedback, and to allow the learner to master a specific task or skill. It can also be combined with role-modeling of new skills by the preceptor that can be practiced by the learner on a new patient at a later time.

## ❖ Learner-Centered Precepting

In the same way skillful clinicians do patient-centered visits, learner-centered precepting relies on the learner initiating interactions to focus their own learning needs. This process can help minimize the discordance between what is being taught and what the learner wants to know (15). Learner-centered precepting uses the same techniques of the Microskills model but begins with the learner deliberately and explicitly defining the question to be addressed. It is similar to patient-centered care that begins with eliciting the patient's agenda and attribution of the problem. Similarly, learner-centered precepting begins with the learner defining the agenda in terms of the learning needs associated with the patient's care. This technique helps you to asses the learner's understanding and to focus the teaching (see Summary of Learner-Centered Precepting in Appendix B on page 159).

An effective model of learner-centered case-based learning was developed at the University of Washington by Pinsky (16). Learners using this model report that it helps them organize their thoughts and decreases the number of learner-preceptor teaching mismatches and preceptors report a better understanding of learners' needs. The Pinksy model begins a patient presentation by the learner with a statement of: "My question is" and proceeds with three parts discussed in the Box 5-9.

The presentation begins and ends with the learner's question to the preceptor. Similar to asking a consultant about a case, the learner begins

---

## Box 5-9. Learning-Centered Precepting

**Identification**

▶ The learner first presents the patient-identifying data, visit status (new or return), and the patient's main concern. At this point, the learner makes a generalized assessment of his or her general teaching need for this specific patient encounter, expressed as "My question is (for example) …about the best medication for this patient's rheumatoid arthritis…"

**Information**

▶ The learner then provides the clinical information that you, as the preceptor, need to know in order to care for the patient, including a concise history, the results of the physical examination's pertinent parts, the most likely diagnosis, and an initial plan.

**Issues**

▶ In the last part, the learner formulates a specific, targeted question, about the knowledge, skills, or logistical information that he or she needs to care for the patient. For example, "Is etanercept a good medication for the patient given the lack of response he has had to the other medications I listed?"

---

with a question that guides the preceptor's teaching. After providing all the patient identification and information needed by the preceptor to understand the case, the learner then reiterates a more nuanced statement of the question. In using this technique, the learner is taught to articulate their questions about the case at the beginning of the case presentation. For example, the learner might report (either inside or outside of the examination room), "I have a question about insulin therapy for Mrs. Smith, a new patient with type 1 diabetes…." and at the end of the presentation, "My question is, should she have intensive insulin therapy using an insulin pump?" A question this sophisticated indicates a higher level of learner knowledge than a question such as "Is a blood sugar of 300 OK?" and helps determine your teaching approach as you listen to the remainder of the presentation. The learner who asks the first question obviously has different teaching needs and capabilities than the second learner. This technique also will give you a starting point for discussion if you disagree with the learner's perception of the case. For example, you might say, "I understand you want to discuss the use of an insulin pump, but first we need to figure out why the sugars are so high." This technique role models the skill of negotiation used by skilled clinicians with patients in setting the agenda for a visit.

"Up-front" identification of the learning issue by the learner is a more active approach and is more work for the learner; thus, unless given a reminder, the learner may not do it consistently. To be effective, learners need to learn how to frame their questions at the beginning of the presentation and be given positive feedback when done correctly. They must realize the wide scope of acceptable questions, including informational ("How do I treat diarrhea caused by Giardia?"); institutional processes ("How do I order a nerve conduction study?"); or time management ("I spent thirty minutes with this patient and I am still only halfway through his list of problems. How do I handle this?"). You must remember to respond to the question during the discussion of the case or to demonstrate or guide the learner toward finding the answer on his or her own. Learning-centered precepting can be combined with the techniques used in the Microskills model described previously and the SNAPPS model discussed below.

## ❖ SNAPPS Model of Learner-Centered Precepting

Another learner-centered model of ambulatory education developed at Case Western Reserve is the SNAPPS model (17). SNAPPS is a mnemonic for a six-step, student-led process that is facilitated by the preceptor:

- **S**ummarize briefly the history and findings
- **N**arrow the differential to two or three possibilities
- **A**nalyze the differential by comparing and contrasting the possibilities

- **P**robe the preceptor by asking questions about uncertainties, difficulties, or alternative approaches
- **P**lan management for the patient's medical issues
- **S**elect a case-related issue for self-directed learning

In the SNAPPs method, the learner uses the mnemonic to help organize the case and set the learning stage for the preceptor (see a summary of the SNAPPS model in Appendix B on page 160). The student is expected to take the lead role in moving through the steps. Initially, this may require support and coaching from the preceptor. Initial student feedback has been positive. They feel capable of taking on an active learning role and identifying their own learning needs; they find SNAPPS intuitive and easy to learn; and they appreciate the opportunity to question the preceptor and follow up with a focused, self-directed learning topic. Preceptors report enjoying teaching the student using SNAPPS and also reported feeling relieved of the pressure to create learning points.

### Summarize Briefly the History and Physical Findings

The learner obtains the history, performs an appropriate focused examination, and presents a concise summary to the preceptor. The case summary should not exceed 50% of the total learning encounter for this case and is generally limited to three minutes or less. Additional information, if needed, can be obtained through direct questioning by the preceptor.

### Narrow the Differential Diagnosis to Two or Three Relevant Possibilities

This step is analogous to the commitment step in the Microskills model. For a new problem, the learner generates a differential diagnosis of two or three most likely possibilities. For exacerbations of chronic illnesses , the learner focuses on why the disease has become active on treatment, and for well visits the learner highlights screening or prevention interventions.

### Analyze the Differential by Comparing and Contrasting the Possibilities

The learner uses historical information and findings from the physical examination to support or refute the entities in the differential diagnosis.

Some learners may combine this step with the first step as each entity in the differential diagnosis is identified and analyzed in turn.

*Probe the Preceptor by Asking Questions about Uncertainties, Difficulties, or Alternative Approaches*
This is the step that is unique in learner-centered precepting. The learner initiates the case discussion by asking the preceptor questions to correct knowledge deficits or clear up areas of confusion rather than being questioned by the preceptor. The learner utilizes the preceptor as an expert consultant. Learners may ask, "What is the blood pressure goal for diabetics?", "What are the risk factors for community-acquired MRSA?", or "How do you listen for a pericardial rub?" The nature and level of sophistication of the questions informs the preceptor of the learner's thought processes and level of knowledge.

*Plan Management for the Patient's Medical Issues*
The learner attempts a management plan by committing to a few interventions. The plan is modified, as needed, by the preceptor with an explanation to the learner.

*Select a Case-Related Issue for Self-Directed Learning*
The learner identifies a learning issue at the end of the case discussion or after seeing the patient with the preceptor. The learner then reads about the issue at the earliest convenient moment. Learners are encouraged to keep track of learning issues by noting them on an index card or personal digital assistant. The preceptor may wish to do the same in order to facilitate follow-up with the learner.

## ❖ Reflection

Reflection is a powerful but seldom used case-based teaching strategy. Reflection moves away from addressing the clinical facts of the case and toward discussions of deeper and often more meaningful content that focuses on the professional development of the learner. Three keys to successful use of reflection in clinical teaching have been identified: being a good role model; gaining the trust of the learners; and having skills to facilitate reflection. Good role models are enthusiastic about medicine, patients, and teaching. They are clinically skillful, have content mastery, and emphasize the psychosocial and social aspects of care. Excellent teachers gain the trust of learners by demonstrating their clinical excellence and concern and support for both learners and patients. Facilitation of reflection depends upon recognizing the "teachable moment" and a willingness to ask deeper, often emotionally laden questions.

Good facilitative technique depends on the ability of the preceptor to pick up on learners' thoughts and emotions and to follow up with an appropriate question (18). Examples include "What did you mean by that?" Or, "You seem concerned about the last patient." Another technique is to repeat back a statement made by the learner, encouraging more thoughtful discussion, such as "You learned something important." It is just as effective to pose a reflective question without the stimulus of a learner comment or emotional response. "So what did this patient teach us?" is an example of a preceptor-initiated reflective question. Experts who facilitate reflection do so in the hope of encouraging discussion that is at a deeper, more complex level associated with higher levels of meaning: the moral, ethical, or professional issues.

A barrier to using reflection is our general uneasiness in exploring emotion, interpersonal relationships, and topics related to professionalism, but the absence of reflection has also been identified as an educational deficiency in clinical training (19).

## ❖ Pitfalls of Case-Based Learning

There are certain pitfalls inherent in case-based teaching that reduce its effectiveness. The most commonly encountered problems include the following:

- Taking over the case
- Asking too many questions
- Not allowing sufficient "wait time"

- Inappropriately giving lectures
- Asking questions with "preprogrammed answers"
- Pushing the learner past his or her ability
- Not giving feedback

*Taking Over the Case*

Taking over the case is one of the most common and educationally destructive pitfalls of case-based learning. Typically, this is most likely to occur when a learner gives an incorrect answer to one of the Microskills questions (e.g., "What do you think is going on?"). Rather than probing further to find what the learner knows or where the learner has gone astray in the diagnostic reasoning process, the preceptor takes control. The learner is told the diagnosis, what investigations to order, medications to prescribe, and any follow-up plans to pursue. At best, the learner becomes a scribe, taking notes to follow up on the preceptor's suggestions and, at worst, becomes a passive bystander with no role in the case management and no opportunity to learn. A corollary of this mistake is not using the encounter to diagnose the learner. This often occurs from a failure to create an environment where the learner feels comfortable expressing his or her own view. Instead, the learner will try to guess what you want to hear; this becomes an effective barrier to diagnosing the learner's knowledge or thinking skills.

*Asking Too Many Questions*

Asking too many questions can lead to learner fatigue and the teaching becoming teacher-centered rather than learner-centered. Asking too many questions may represent an unconscious attempt to display breadth of knowledge or avoid answering the learner's questions. Try to reflect after a teaching episode on who was controlling the conversation, and, thereby, the learning, and whether or not this was in the best interest of the learner.

*Not Allowing Sufficient "Wait Time"*

Closely related to taking over the case is not allowing sufficient "wait time" when asking the learner a question. Physicians have a tendency, whether dealing with patients or learners, to interrupt and ask another question or provide the answer to the first question when an answer is not immediately forthcoming. Having discovered that impatience discourages any real attempt on the part of the learner to answer the question, effective teachers allow the learner more time to consider the question and to formulate a response. When preceptors answer their own questions, learners are quick to recognize that they are not really expected to answer the question and do not put forth the effort. Alternatively, learners working with patient preceptors who wait for an answer learn not only that an answer is expected—even if it is wrong—but also that it is an essential and expected component of the learning process.

### Inappropriately Giving Lectures

Another common problem with case-based learning is giving lectures inappropriately when the learner can independently gather information with greater educational impact at a later time. As presented in the Microskills model, teaching can be given in small "bites" of information. These small "bites" include teaching a general rule and relating it to the immediate situation. For example, "For most young, healthy individuals with back pain, ordering a back X-ray is not cost effective; therefore, we will not order it for Mr. Smith. He fits the profile of patients who do not benefit from an X-ray." The learner can be directed to the primary information sources that support this general rule, and any follow-up reading can be done at a later time. The primary data supporting the general rule should not be presented by you in the form of a mini-lecture.

### Asking Questions with "Preprogrammed Answers"

As suggested in the Microskills section, preceptors must learn not to ask questions with "preprogrammed answers" that immediately suggest the correct answer, thereby preventing any thinking on part of the learner. An example of a question with a "preprogrammed answer" is "What do you think is going on? Could it be gastritis?" The answer is obvious; it requires no problem solving or data synthesis on part of the learner, and it deprives you of the ability to assess the learner's knowledge and problem-solving skills.

*Pushing the Learner Past His or Her Ability*

Another common problem with case-based learning is pushing the learner past his or her ability. This usually takes the form of discussing the ramifications of a case beyond his or her comprehension of what is being said or asked. An example would be asking a learner about the advantages of using an angiotensin-converting–enzyme inhibitor in a hypertensive patient with diabetes when he or she has not yet learned about diabetic nephropathy. The key to knowing you have pushed beyond the learner's ability is observing the reaction to your question. Lack of response, lack of follow-up questions, or a neutral facial expression typically signal incomprehension. At this point, the best strategy is assessing what the learner does know by using probing questions. Do not ask questions that can be answered with a simple "yes" or "no" (e.g., "Do you know what diabetic nephropathy is?"); ask questions that require the learner to explain and synthesize information (e.g., "What do you recall about the effects diabetes has on the kidney?").

The following illustrates a series of probing questions that can help assess the learner's grasp of content:

- "What is the relationship between long-standing hyper-glycemia and kidney function?"
- "What is the proposed mechanism?"
- "How can it be prevented?"

*Not Giving Feedback*

Corrective and positive feedback change behavior but is rarely done in clinical teaching (see Learner Feedback and Evaluation in Chapter 8). Certain opportunities are ripe for feedback and should be exploited whenever possible. Examples include commenting on an empathic dialog between learner and patient, well-organized case presentations, provision of culturally sensitive patient education, incorporation of previous feedback into practice, and evidence of independent reading. Some feedback is better than none, and it does not need to be extensive in order to be helpful.

The following are examples of short, positive feedback statements that will encourage the learner to persist with the desired behavior:

- "I liked the way you reassured the patient. She was less anxious and able to concentrate on your instructions."
- "Your case presentation was excellent, concise but containing all the relevant information."
- "I see that you remembered how to listen for an $S_3$; this will help you diagnose heart failure."

## ❖ Concluding the Visit

Regardless of the teaching model used, take time at the end of the visit to review with the learner his or her follow-up responsibilities. These might include the following tasks:

- Arranging for a follow-up appointment, consultation, imaging study, or laboratory work
- Performing vaccinations and other health-maintenance and screening procedures
- Educating patients
- Writing or dictating a chart note
- Updating the "Problem List," "Medication List," and "Health Maintenance/Screening Form"
- Finding data absent from the chart (e.g., laboratory work, consultation, previous note)
- Making "to do" notes (e.g., follow-up telephone call with patient)
- Taking on an independent learning assignment, if appropriate

You might make a note of the patients seen by the learner. This will remind you to follow up with the learner on such things as laboratory results, consultations, and results of therapeutic interventions. Such notes could be kept on a copy of the daily schedule and saved as a patient log for you and the learner. Viewed over time, this information is also useful in determining the adequacy of the learner's experience in terms of numbers of patients seen and their medical and social diversity. It also will help remind you of things the learner has done well and other incidents when you are completing the end-of-rotation evaluation.

## REFERENCES

1. **Neher JO, Gordon KC, Meyer B, Stevens N.** A five-step "microskills" model of clinical teaching. J Am Board Fam Prac. 1992;5:419-24.
2. **Whitman NA, Schwenk TL.** Preceptors as Teachers. Salt Lake City, UT: University of Utah School of Medicine; 1984.
3. **Loftus TH, McLeod PJ, Snell LS.** Faculty perceptions of effective ambulatory care teaching. J Gen Intern Med. 1993;8:575-7.
4. **McGee SR, Irby DM.** Teaching in the outpatient clinic: practical tips. J Gen Intern Med. 1997;12(Suppl):S34-40.
5. **Furney SL, Orsini AN, Orsetti KE, et al.** Teaching the one-minute preceptor. A randomized controlled trial. J Gen Intern Med. 2001;16:620-4.
6. **Aagaard E, Teherani A, Irby DM.** Effectiveness of the one-minute preceptor model for diagnosing the patient and the learner: proof of concept. Acad Med. 2004;79:42-9.
7. **Salerno SM, O'Malley PG, Pangaro LN, et al.** Faculty development seminars based on the one-minute preceptor improve feedback in the ambulatory setting. J Gen Intern Med. 2002;17:779-87.
8. **Irby DM, Aagaard E, Teherani A.** Teaching points identified by preceptors observing one-minute preceptor and traditional preceptor encounters. Acad Med. 2004;79:50-5.
9. **Wilkerson L, Armstrong E, Lesky L.** Faculty development for ambulatory teaching. J Gen Intern Med. 1990;5(Suppl):S44-53.
10. **Skeff KM.** Enhancing teaching effectiveness and vitality in the ambulatory setting. J Gen Intern Med. 1988;3(Suppl):S26-33.
11. **Cunningham AS, Blatt SD, Fuller PG, Weinberger HL.** The art of precepting: Socrates or Aunt Minnie? Arch Pediatr Adolesc Med. 1999;153:114-6.
12. **Sackett DL, Haynes RB, Tugwell P.** Clinical Epidemiology: A Basic Science for Clinical Medicine, 1st ed. Boston: Little, Brown; 1985.
13. **Heidenreich C, Lye P, Simpson D, Lourich M.** The search for effective and efficient ambulatory teaching methods through the literature. Pediatrics. 2000;105:231-7.
14. **Ferenchick G, Simpson D, Blackman J, et al.** Strategies for efficient and effective teaching in the ambulatory care setting. Acad Med. 1997;72:277-80.
15. **Laidley TL, Braddock CH, Fihn SD.** Did I answer your question? Attending physicians' recognition of residents' perceived learning needs in ambulatory settings. J Gen Intern Med. 2000;15:46-50.
16. **Pinsky L.** 'My question is...'—learner-centered precepting. Med Educ. 2003;37:486-7.
17. **Wolpaw TM, Wolpaw DR, Papp KK.** SNAPPS: a learner-centered model for outpatient education. Acad Med. 2003;78:893-8.
18. **Branch WT Jr, Paranjape A.** Feedback and reflection: teaching methods for clinical settings. Acad Med. 2002;77:1185-8.
19. **Coulehan J, Williams PC.** Vanquishing virtue: the impact of medical education. Acad Med. 2001;76:598-605.

# 6

# Ways to Be More Efficient When Teaching

This chapter presents eight strategies that can be used to become more efficient or to make up lost time in the office, namely:

- The Focused Half Day
- Presenting in the Room
- Collaborative Examinations
- Active Observation
- Dual Teaching
- Service-Based Education
- Just-in-Time Learning
- Self-Directed (Independent) Learning

## ❖ The Focused Half Day

The focused half day is a useful and efficient teaching strategy suggested by Taylor and colleagues at the Medical College of Ohio (1). This method has its greatest value when precepting clinically inexperienced learners. You and the learner begin by reviewing the patient schedule, either the night before or at the very beginning of the session. You use this opportunity to review the reason for each patient's visit. After the entire list is reviewed, you and the learner pick a "teaching issue" for the day and select a limited number of patients that address the teaching issue. The patient schedule becomes the "table of contents" for that day's learning. The theme of the teaching issue can be disease based (for example, diabetes), a procedural skill (taking blood pressures), related to the history (taking a sexual history) or the physical examination (liver palpation). Learners are given time before seeing the selected patients to prepare for the encounter by reviewing the patient's chart or reading about the selected teaching issue for that day. This specific activity of preparation and reflection gives the learner a meaningful task while you are pursuing other office-related activities, reducing the learner's "down-time" that learners often complain about.

Early experience with the focused half day model is positive (1). First-year students report that this organizing strategy is extremely beneficial, and preceptors found it helpful and practical. Preceptors commented that it helped them know "where students were coming from," and enhanced their confidence as teachers.

## ❖ Presenting in the Room

Traditionally, learners report their findings to the teacher outside of the examination room. If you use this model, the next step involves returning to the room to verify the history and physical examination and to plan the care for the patient. A time-saving step would be to have the learner present the patient's case in the examining room in front of the patient. Due to concerns of patient acceptance, preceptors have not adopted this technique universally. However, studies of in-the-room presentations by residents and students in both the in-patient and ambulatory setting show that patients actually approve of and prefer this strategy. Patients report that, with "bed-side" presentations (in this case, inside the examination room), doctors spent more time with them and offered better explanations of their problems. Such presentations did not provoke worry, and patients were satisfied with the overall process (2-5). Patients with in-room presentations by medical students were more likely to report that the student was a greater contribution to the patient's satisfaction (5). It is important, however, that the learner alert you of any potentially sensitive issues or serious diagnoses being considered before making the presentation. As always, these issues must be handled with care and sensitivity. The learners must be told this and be aware of the power of their words.

When using in-the-room presentations, take time to introduce the concept to the patient (6). You may begin by saying, "I hope it is all right if the student/resident tells me what you have been talking about. It is my job not to interrupt. When she/he finishes, I will ask you if anything was missed or if you have something to add and then we will talk about what to do." This useful statement accomplishes a number of important tasks. First, it asks permission to proceed, sets the expectation of not interrupting, and tells the patient they will have a chance to add information or clarify points. You may also want to give the patient permission to interrupt if you say something they don't understand. You can tell the patient that "doctors have been trained to communicate with each other in medical terms and may mistakenly fall back into this habit, but we do not mean to exclude you from the conversation." By stating this to the patient, you concurrently reassure the patient and remind the learner not to use jargon.

Despite high patient acceptance and the obvious time-saving benefits for you, not all learners are comfortable presenting in the room (3,4), and they may have to be convinced of its value. Interestingly, students who are consistently asked to present in the room report a small preference for in-room presentations, compared to students who do not routinely present in the room, suggesting that frequent use decreases learner apprehension (5). Some of the benefits of presenting in the room include the following:

- It saves time
- Patients perceive in-the-room presentations as being more confidential than "hallway talk"
- Patients are not waiting alone for the doctors

- Patients prefer to hear what is being said about them
- Learners tend to make more concise presentations
- Patients can verify information
- Patients can correct misinformation
- It increases the preceptor's "face-to-face" time with the patient
- The preceptor can immediately collect additional information that flows naturally from the learner's presentation
- Patients feel they are part of the process
- It helps maintain compliance with the Health Care Financing Administration (HCFA) regulations on billing for services that need to be performed personally by the physician

Despite the enthusiasm of most patients and preceptors about in-the-room presentations, not all discussion between the preceptor and learner should be in front of the patient. Analyzing the learner's thought processes or discussing the differential diagnosis are more suited for private conversations, particularly if they are likely to include entities that are emotionally charged. Discussions of pathophysiology or debates about the literature are best reserved for out-of-room presentations.

Notwithstanding reassurances about the educational value and efficiency of bedside presentations, some learners will be resistant. In these cases, we suggest that you encourage in-room presentations as they are good opportunities to role model clinical skills and to involve patients in the decision-making process. This may be your best opportunity to demonstrate empathy, compassion, and concern and to validate the usefulness of a skillfully taken history and a focused examination. If this strategy works for you, simply make it happen.

## ❖ Collaborative Examinations

Collaborative examinations involve the learner and preceptor seeing the patient simultaneously. This technique is most time efficient when working with students. The student takes the lead in taking the history, with you observing. The student is given a defined amount of time to accomplish the task. After the student has completed the history, you can ask any additional questions, with the student observing. Then, the student can be assigned certain parts of the examination to be performed under your direct observation, followed by you repeating parts of the examination to verify essential findings. This technique is useful when attempting to gauge a new learner's level of expertise. It also can be used when formally evaluating a learner or simply to save time. Finally, collaborative examinations offer an excellent opportunity to role model clinical skills and, like presenting in the room, help maintain compliance with the HCFA regulations on billing for services that need to be performed personally by the physician.

### ❖ Active Observation

Active observation is a useful technique for both students and residents when time is a factor or when the complexity of the problem is too sophisticated for the learner (see Summary of Active Observation in Appendix B on page 161). In active observation, the learner is asked to observe you performing a clinical skill. The skill may be communication, interviewing, physical examination, or procedural.

*Active Observation Is Not Shadowing*
Care must be taken not to transform this exercise into mere "shadowing," which makes the learner a passive participant. Observation can become an active learning process by "priming" the learner, i.e., describing what will happen, why it needs to happen, and what to look for. Follow up the session with an opportunity for the learner to describe what happened and to practice what was just learned. For active observation to be effective, the following must occur:
- The learner needs to be informed about the rationale for the observation. Example: "This patient is very hostile, and I want you to watch how I manage this situation."
- The learner should be told what to observe. Example: "Notice how I diffuse his anger by labeling and validating his emotions."

- The learner should be provided with an opportunity to review what was learned after the session. Example: "Tell me what you saw when I interviewed the patient."

The learner should be observed practicing what was taught and should be provided feedback on his or her performance. In one study of students, 70% responded that active observation was the most important learning event in their ambulatory medicine rotation (7). See Box 6-1 for a summary of the critical elements in active observation.

---

**Box 6-1. Summary of the Critical Elements in Active Observation**

▶ Describing the rationale for the observation ("You should watch me do this because...")

▶ Declaring what the learner should observe ("Watch how I ...")

▶ Reviewing what was observed ("What did you see happen in that session?")

▶ Allowing the learner an opportunity to practice ("When you see the next patient, I want you to...")

---

### ❖ Dual Teaching

Dual teaching is a strategy commonly used by experienced preceptors to improve efficiency (8). Dual teaching means providing health education to a patient simultaneously while teaching or assesing the student. There are a number of variants of the strategy. In the first variant you assume the educator's role and direct the short, relevant educational message to either the student or the patient. The essential point is that both student and patient are present when the message is delevered and both benefit. In a second variant, the learner takes on the educator's role and you observe, ready to provide feedback outside of the room at the end of the session. This works particularly well if the learner had previously observed you performing this task. You can assess the learner's mastery of the content, communication skills and interpersonal style. Once proficient in this task, the learner can deliver the educational message to the patient alone, freeing you or your office staff for other tasks (see Service-Based Education, below).

## ❖ Service-Based Education

Service-based education can be an effective teaching strategy for students. It consists of identifying tasks that typically are performed by a member of the office staff (or occasionally by you) and training the student to perform those tasks (9). This is not to suggest that service-based education can replace the clinical encounter as the main focus of office-based teaching, rather it is meant to supplement the clinical encounter. The advantages to the learner are 1) the opportunity to gain knowledge about and perform tasks that are often critical to the efficient operation of an office and 2) to develop a sense of being a contributing member of the office team. The benefits to the office can be significant, e.g., a student may be able to "free up" a member of the office staff for a period of time to accomplish other tasks. Some of the tasks that students can perform while in the office setting include the following:

- Counseling and education of patients
- Diabetic foot exams (e.g., using a template)
- Retrieving laboratory or radiology results
- Making follow-up telephone calls
- Triaging patient calls
- Filling out laboratory, radiology, and consultation request forms
- Administering vaccinations
- Conducting patients to the examination room, documenting the reason for the visit, recording vital signs
- Performing electrocardiography and other simple office laboratory tests
- Chart audits for quality improvement
- Answering clinical questions by using databases (e.g., PubMed)

The main idea behind service-based education is not to reduce your office overhead by taking advantage of the student's services but rather to introduce the student to the tasks, talents, and time necessary to run an office. Some of the tasks (e.g., filing and retrieving charts) may require only an hour or two to accomplish, whereas others (e.g., triaging patient telephone calls) may require several hours of dedicated time to capture the complexity and importance of the task. In any event, service-based education is a supplement to, not a replacement of, clinical encounters and patient-based learning.

## ❖ Just-in-Time Learning

Between patients, you can quickly review learning issues related to a patient just seen (10). If you have used the Microskills or one of the learner-centered teaching models, you have probably identified a learning need that is suited for practicing evidence-based medicine skills. Ask the learner to formulate a clinical question and, time allowing, look up the answer using your favorite sources of evidence-based information (for example, POEMs, Evidence-Based Medicine for Primary Care and Internal Medicine, ACP Physician Information and Education Resource, the *ACP Journal Club*, or Cochrane Library). Have the learner begin this task as you see the next patient alone, allowing you to catch up in your schedule if you are falling behind. This "catch up" strategy is particularly useful when working with inexperienced learners. This strategy is valuable for the student as well; integrating evidence-based medicine into practice in this fashion is one of the top three factors students associate with effective teaching (11).

## ❖ Self-Directed (Independent) Learning

When there is a lull in the office (e.g., lunch time, end of the day), ask the learner a few questions that stimulate reflection and promote self-directed learning (12-14) (see Summary of Self-Directed [Independent Learning] in Appendix B on page 162). Such questions might include the following:

- "Based on the patients you saw today, what are your questions?"
- "What did you learn today?"
- "What was the most important thing that happened today?"
- "What is the one thing you would like to learn more about?"
- "What troubled you today?"
- "What might you improve on?"

Considering role modeling this behavior by indicating what you learned today, what questions were generated for you, and how you intend to answer them. By role modeling the behavior, you demonstrate the importance of this approach to continuing education. You also can use this time to ask the learner to participate in some self-directed learning.

The two essential steps in self-directed learning are the identification of the limits of one's knowledge and skills and the ability to organize resources to learn more (15). Self-directed study engages the learner in critical thinking and hands-on experiences that promote application of book knowledge to "real world" experiences. Self-directed learning also can promote the study of diseases and conditions that the learner is unlikely to see at the office due to case mix and prevalence.

To maximize effectiveness, self-directed learning should be linked to a recently observed patient problem. The opportunity to store knowledge in the context from which it will be retrieved (i.e., case-based learning) aids the learning process (16). Additionally, reading around recently encountered cases is more motivating than asking learners to tackle the textbook chapter by chapter.

Self-directed learning is a reasonable learning goal for either the student or resident. If learning resources are available in the office, learners can be asked to pursue questions that remain unanswered after a patient visit, with the understanding that the information will be conveyed back to you at a later but specifically defined time. For example, a convenient review time might be at the end of the day after all the patients have been seen. Also, asking the learner to pursue unanswered questions through independent reading is a technique that can be used to help you "catch up" when you are behind in your schedule. While the learner is reading, you can see one or two patients independently.

Box 6-2 summarizes the main components of self-directed learning; this can be used as a checklist when making assignments for learners in the office:

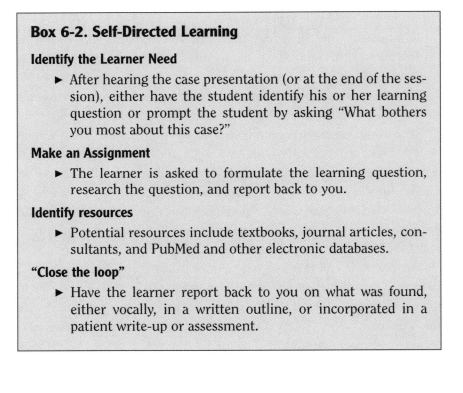

**Box 6-2. Self-Directed Learning**

**Identify the Learner Need**

▶ After hearing the case presentation (or at the end of the session), either have the student identify his or her learning question or prompt the student by asking "What bothers you most about this case?"

**Make an Assignment**

▶ The learner is asked to formulate the learning question, research the question, and report back to you.

**Identify resources**

▶ Potential resources include textbooks, journal articles, consultants, and PubMed and other electronic databases.

**"Close the loop"**

▶ Have the learner report back to you on what was found, either vocally, in a written outline, or incorporated in a patient write-up or assessment.

The educational prescription is a tool that can help both you and the learner formalize the process of self-directed learning (see Educational Prescription Form in Appendix A on page 131).

## REFERENCES

1. **Taylor C, Lipsky MS, Bauer L.** Focused teaching: facilitating early clinical experience in an office setting. Fam Med. 1998;30:547-8.
2. **Lehmann LS, Brancati FL, Chen MC, et al.** The effect of bedside case presentations on patient's perceptions of their medical care. N Engl J Med. 1997;336:1150-5.
3. **Wang-Cheng RM, Barnas GP, Sigmann P, et al.** Bedside case presentations: why patients like them but learners don't. J Gen Intern Med. 1989;4:284-7.
4. **Anderson RJ, Cyran E, Schilling L, et al.** Outpatient case presentations in the conference room versus examination room: results from two randomized controlled trials. Am J Med. 2002;113:657-62.
5. **Rogers HD, Carline JD, Paauw DS.** Examination room presentations in general internal medicine clinic: patients' and students' perceptions. Acad Med. 2003;78:945-9.
6. **DeWitt DE.** Incorporating medical students into your practice. Aust Fam Physician. 2006;35:24-6.
7. **Epstein RM, Cole DR, Gawinski BA, et al.** How students learn from community-based preceptors. Arch Fam Med. 1998;7:149-54.
8. **Usatine RP, Tremoulet PT, Irby D.** Time-efficient preceptors in ambulatory care settings. Acad Med. 2000;75:639-42.
9. **Regan-Smith M, Young WW, Keller AM.** An efficient and effective teaching model for ambulatory education. Acad Med. 2002;77:593-9.
10. **Dobbie AE, Tysinger JW, Freeman J.** Strategies for efficient office precepting. Fam Med. 2005;37:239-41.
11. **Elnicki DM, Kolarik R, Bardella I.** Third-year medical students' perceptions of effective teaching behaviors in a multidisciplinary ambulatory clerkship. Acad Med. 2003;78: 815-9.
12. **Arseneau R.** Exit rounds: a reflection exercise. Acad Med. 1995;70:684-87.
13. **DaRosa DA, Dunningham GL, Stearns J, et al.** Ambulatory teaching "lite": less clinic time, more educationally fulfilling. Acad Med. 1997;72:358-61.
14. **Smith CS, Irby DM.** The roles of experience and reflection in ambulatory care education. Acad Med. 1997;72:32-5.
15. **Skeff KM.** Enhancing teaching effectiveness and vitality in the ambulatory setting. J Gen Intern Med. 1988;3(Suppl):S26-33.
16. **Bordage G.** Elaborated knowledge: a key to successful diagnostic thinking. Acad Med. 1994;70:883-5.

# 7

# Teaching Procedures in the Office

Many patients expect their physician to perform needed procedures. However, surveys of trainees indicate that many do not feel confident in performing common ambulatory procedures, citing inadequate training (1-4). Teaching procedures in an academic medical center can be problematic. Barriers include lack of trained faculty, adequate patient numbers, cost, and access to equipment (5,6). Community practices offer a viable alternative to the academic medical center, but in order to be efficient and effective and to ensure patient safety, a systematic approach to procedural training should be followed. The remainder of this chapter is based on one systematic approach developed by Stephen Yelon, PhD, Professor Emeritus of the Department of Counseling, Special Education and Educational Psychology, Michigan State University (7,8). For the purposes of this chapter we will focus on a process to teach procedural skills with the understanding that the same approach is applicable to teaching all types of skills, including physical examination and communication skills.

### ❖ Knowing the Skill Through and Through

In order to teach a skill effectively, you must develop an unconscious awareness of the skill so you can explain it, demonstrate it, and evaluate the learners' performance. Unconscious awareness of a skill can develop as the result of repeated performances to the point that the execution of the steps and their proper sequencing becomes automatic. This part of the process is already mastered by experienced clinicians interested in teaching procedural skills. The difficult part is the detailed analysis of the skill and its subsequent articulation as individual steps and sub-steps. The final product of a detailed skill analysis is the creation of a set of written learning objectives and a checklist of the skill's steps in their proper sequence.

### ❖ Creating Learning Objectives

The creation of learning objectives may seem like unnecessary "busy work" but the effort pays dividends in the long run. Learning objectives help clarify for you and the learner what you are trying to accomplish. Detailed learning objectives outline for the learner exact expectations and criteria for successful performance. Yelon has proposed creating learning objectives (7,8), and based on his advice we suggest an objective that addresses the identification of the skill, performance situations, qualities defining good performance, desired results, and indications of proficiency (see Box 7-1).

---

### Box 7-1. Example of Learning Objectives for Shave Biopsy

**Skill:** Perform shave biopsy

**Situation:** Adult patient with exophytic lesions

**Qualities defining good performance:** Obtaining informed consent; identification and collection of equipment and supplies; follow universal precautions; proper cleansing of biopsy site; adequate anesthesia; stabilization of the skin; superficial shave; establishing hemostasis; proper handling of the specimen; dressing the wound; articulation of post-procedure patient instructions.

*continued*

---

> **Results:** Informed consent properly obtained; patient comfort is maintained; universal precautions observed; procedure performed smoothly and efficiently; bleeding is controlled; specimen identified and sent to laboratory; wound is dressed; follow up instructions are provided.
>
> **Indicators of proficiency:** Shave biopsy performed properly 3 out of 3 times on an adult without mistake.

The creation of the skill-based learning objectives relies heavily on your judgment and past experience as an expert in performing the skill.

## ❖ Creating a Skill Checklist

Equally important as the learning objectives is the written analysis (description) of the skill. A completed analysis will allow you to quickly identify the prerequisites, steps and sub-steps, and the proper sequencing of the steps. It has been our experience that it often takes three or four iterations before we are satisfied that all component steps are described and arranged in their proper sequence. It is a good idea to give the written analysis to a colleague with the question, "Could you perform this procedure simply by following these instructions?" This type of review can quickly identify any absent steps, ambiguities, or incorrect sequencing. From the written analysis you can create a skill checklist to function as a teaching and learning aid and an evaluation document. You can use the checklist while teaching the procedure as a reminder of the steps and their sequence. This prevents you from skipping over steps that are automatic for you but unknown to the learner. The learner can use the checklist to help memorize the steps and to aid independent practice. Finally, when observing the learner performing the skill, the checklist aids you in recording performance and providing feedback. See Box 7-2 for an example of a skill checklist for a shave biopsy. For conciseness, this checklist was abbreviated to focus only on the performance steps of the procedure itself.

**Box 7-2. Shave Biopsy Checklist**

**Prepare the Site**
► Clean the site with alcohol or chlorhexidine gluconate

**Anesthetize the Skin**
► Position the needle perpendicular to the skin
► Inject intradermally
► Raise a wheal under the lesion

**Stabilize the Skin**
► Stretch the skin with the finger and thumb

**Select Cutting Instrument**
► Razor or #15 scalpel

**Make Incision**
► Angle scalpel blade or curve razor between thumb and forefinger for proper depth
► Use a smooth cutting motion directed parallel to the stabilizing thumb and forefinger

**Secure the Specimen**
► Place specimen in a 10% buffered formalin
► Label specimen container (patient name and biopsy location)

**Establish Hemostasis**
► Apply firm pressure to wound with gauze pad
► Apply aluminum chloride to dry wound base

**Dress Wound**
► Cover wound with petrolatum and adhesive dressing

## ❖ The Introductory Phase

When teaching a new skill, begin by motivating the learner. Often, this will not be necessary because the request to learn the skill comes directly from the learner who is already motivated and anxious to learn. In the absence of self-motivating behavior, tell the learner why the skill is important, how it can be used, and its significance to you and your patients. Relate the skill to "real-world" practical performance. For example, you might say, "Dermatology accounts for over 30% of my practice. Many of my older patients have exophytic skin lesions that need to be removed to either confirm a diagnosis or provide definitive treatment and they prefer to have the procedure done in the office rather than be referred out. Being competent in this procedure provides a needed service for my patients and is also another source of income to help meet my overhead."

Next, you can explore what the learner already knows. This prevents you from teaching skills that have already been mastered by the learner and allows you to concentrate on the deficiencies. For example, the learner may be unfamiliar with a shave biopsy but may have extensive experience in local anesthesia acquired during an emergency department rotation. Of course, it is always best to confirm first hand what the learner knows and what they can do before finalizing your teaching script.

Armed with the knowledge of what the leaner already knows, provide a concise overview of the skill along with the learning objectives. During the overview, review only essential information, progressively filling in the finer details later during the demonstration and practice sessions. For example, an overview of the shave biopsy might be presented as, "A shave biopsy is a common and simple office technique that uses either a scalpel or ordinary razor blade to remove growths from the surface of the skin. It is a clean, not a sterile, technique and doesn't require suturing. There are six major steps: preparing the site, achieving anesthesia, shaving the lesion, establishing hemostasis, securing the specimen, and dressing the wound."

After the overview, demonstrate the skill. This can be done on a patient after informing the patient of your intent and obtaining permission. Focus the learner on what to observe. Provide the learner with the skill checklist so he/she can follow the important steps. While demonstrating the procedure for the learner, name each step out loud in its proper order as it is performed. Focus on correct performance and indicators of quality for the essential steps, basing them on your past experience. For example, you might say, "I know that I have injected the anesthetic correctly when I see a wheal develop beneath the lesion that is about 2 mm high, like a big mosquito bite." If it is not possible to immediately demonstrate the skill on a patient, consider using diagrams or video demonstrations instead. Many common office procedures are now introduced to learners using video; check with your sponsoring institution to see if these are available for your use. Video demonstrations help the learner conceptualize the application of theoretical knowledge and can be reviewed in whole or in part many times until the learner becomes familiar with the content (9,10). Visual images in combination with verbal instruction have also been shown to significantly increase recall and retention (9).

After you have demonstrated the skill, ask the learner to commit the checklist steps to memory. Begin by reviewing the steps again with the learner then have the learner use the checklist to recite the steps alone and finally silently recite each step and visualize performing them. The process of memorizing the steps may take the learner 10 or 15 minutes and can be done while you are engaged in another task. Creating one-word "code" names for each of the steps might help the learner quickly memorize the steps. For example you can represent each of the major steps in the shave biopsy with the following memorization aids:

- Clean (Prepare the site with alcohol or chlorhexidine gluconate)
- Stab (Anesthetize the skin)
- Stretch (Stabilize the skin)
- Pick (Select cutting instrument)
- Shave (make incision)
- Plop (Secure the specimen in formalin)
- Press (Establish hemostatis with pressure)
- Dab (Apply aluminum chloride to wound)
- Slop (Cover wound with petrolatum)
- Slap (Cover wound with adhesive dressing)

Check back with the learner after this stage is completed to verify that the steps are memorized.

## ❖ The Practice Phase

This phase involves the learner practicing the skill under your direct observation. You may wish to have the learner first practice in a simulated situation. Local anesthetic (saline for practice) can be injected into an orange peal, allowing the learner get over the initial awkwardness of handling unfamiliar tools and performing new tasks such as drawing up fluid into a small syringe, holding the syringe at the proper angle, and manipulating the plunger. A shave biopsy can be practiced scores of time on a pig's foot (available from the grocery store) and practice improves the learner's psychomotor skills and boosts confidence before attempting the procedure on a patient. Furthermore, simulated practice opportunities allow the learner to practice independently until comfortable with all the steps in their proper order. At the time the learner indicates readiness, you can watch the learner perform a simulated procedure and use the checklist to verify sufficient mastery of the steps to perform the procedure on a patient under your supervision. Before going to the patient, remind the trainees not to say "oops" in front of a patient if they make a mistake and review other ways to respond.

When moving to a patient, explain to the patient what will happen and reassure the patient you will be right there guiding the learner. Answer the patient's questions, address their concerns, and obtain their consent before proceeding. It is been our experience that most patients are happy to be involved in a teaching exercise of this nature, particularly if they are made a partner in the learning experience.

Whether practicing on a simulator or on a patient, you can provide moment-to-moment prompts to coach the learner's performance. Whenever possible, use reflection to reinforce the learning. For example, if the learner is about to perform a shave without stabilizing the skin, you might stop the learner and ask, "What do you remember about stabilizing the skin?" At the end of the procedure, review with the learner what was done well, what needs to improve, and steps to take to get next level of performance. Remember to be flexible when you observe deviations from the stated protocol if, in your judgment, they are not important and not associated with an adverse outcome.

## ❖ The Perfecting Phase

This phase is an opportunity for the learner to practice the skill in multiple different situations in order to consolidate the learning. Prior to performing the procedure, ask the learner to engage in mental practice, visualizing performing the procedure with all the requisite steps. During the perfecting phase, provide the learner with many realistic and progressively difficult situations. Using the shave biopsy as an example, this might include performing the procedure on different parts of the body, removing larger lesions, removing multiple lesions in one setting, or performing the procedure on a patient taking aspirin or warfarin. During this phase continue to observe, prompt, and give feedback. It is during the perfecting phase that you go beyond the essential components of the procedure and begin to elaborate on the finer points. This might include how to modify the depth of the shave depending on the nature of the lesion or how to manage recalcitrant bleeding. The learner is more apt to focus and learn these finer points once they have mastered the essential steps. Presenting the finer points too early in the process can impede the efficient learning of the basic steps. (See Box 7-3 and Teaching Procedural Skills in this chapter on for a summary of essential steps.)

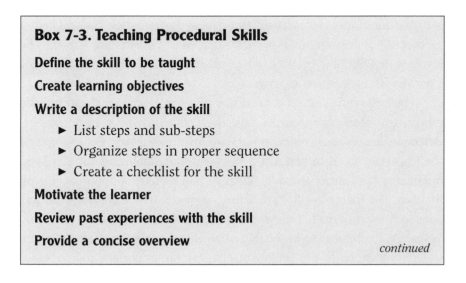

**Box 7-3. Teaching Procedural Skills**

**Define the skill to be taught**

**Create learning objectives**

**Write a description of the skill**

  ▶ List steps and sub-steps

  ▶ Organize steps in proper sequence

  ▶ Create a checklist for the skill

**Motivate the learner**

**Review past experiences with the skill**

**Provide a concise overview**

*continued*

**Demonstrate the skill**
- ► Name each essential step as it is performed
- ► Focus on correct performance and quality indicators

**Commit steps to memory (consider using code names for each step)**

**Practice (simulation first, if possible)**
- ► Observe and prompt learner
- ► Provide feedback

**Perfecting**
- ► Provide increasingly difficult or different practice situations
- ► Elaborate finer points

**Document proficiency**

## REFERENCES

1. **Wickstrom GC, Kolar MM, Keyserling TC, et al.** Confidence of graduating internal medicine residents to perform ambulatory procedures. J Gen Intern Med 2000;15:361-65.
2. **Wickstrom GC, Kelley DK, Keyserling TC, et al.** Confidence of academic general internists and family physicians to teach ambulatory procedures. J Gen Intern Med 2000;15:353-60.
3. **Mandel JH, Rich EC, Luxenberg MG, Spilane MT, Kern DC, Parrino TA.** Preparation for practice in internal medicine: a study of ten years of residency graduates. Arch Intern Med 1988;148:853-56.
4. **Kern DC, Parrino TA, Korst DR.** The lasting value of clinical skills. JAMA 1985;254:70-76.
5. **Norris TE, Cullison SW, Fihn SD.** Teaching Procedural Skills. J Gen Intern Med 1997;12:S64-70.
6. **Sierpina VS, Volk RJ.** Teaching outpatient procedures: most common settings, evaluation methods, and training barriers in family practice residencies. Fam Med 1998;30:421-23.
7. **Yelon SL.** Powerful Principles of Instruction. White Plains (NY): Longman Publishers; 1996.
8. **Yelon SL.** Goal Oriented Instructional Design. East Lansing (MI); SLY Publishers; 2002.
9. **Dwyer FM.** Strategies for improving visual learning. State College, PA: Learning Services;1978.
10. **MacKinney AA.** On teaching beside diagnostic and therapeutic procedures to medical students: an annotated bibliography of audiovisual materials. J Gen Intern Med 1994;9:153-57.

# Learner Feedback and Evaluation

This chapter addresses the relationship between assessment, feedback, and evaluation. It presents useful tips on how to provide effective feedback and systematically evaluate a learner, describes a useful evaluation model, and summarizes how to avoid evaluation errors.

## ❖ What Is Feedback and Why Is It Important?

Feedback is an essential part of helping learners improve and is the most commonly cited "teaching" method described in the literature (1). It is based on your first-hand assessment of the learner's knowledge, attitude, and skills. Feedback describes appropriate or inappropriate actions or behaviors and thereby provides information (feedback) to learners about their current performance that guides their future learning and performance (2-4).

Learners greatly desire and value feedback (5). The complaint heard most frequently from learners is that no one tells them how they are doing. Learners do not make errors on purpose; most errors that persist are the result of insufficient feedback. Specific feedback is important because it changes behavior. For example, intensive feedback provided to residents significantly improves satisfaction ratings from patients as compared with residents not receiving feedback (6). Ideally, feedback should be given every time you interact with a learner, but realistically this is seldom possible. At a minimum, you should offer feedback at regular intervals during the learning experience.

## ❖ What Are the Different Types of Feedback?

For the office-based preceptor, two different types of feedback are commonly used: brief feedback and formal feedback (7). Brief feedback is the kind you might give as you quickly demonstrate a better physical examination technique or improve a learner's case presentation. It is spontaneous, short, and to the point, e.g., "This is how I listen for a carotid bruit" or "Remember to begin your presentations with the patient's name, age, and reason why she is being seen today." If this brief teaching interaction is preceded by, "Let me give you some feedback," the learner's sensitivity to the instruction is heightened. Brief feedback should be given liberally so that recieving feedback is normalized.

Formal feedback is a planned feedback session, often scheduled at the middle and end of clinical rotations or ambulatory blocks and may be best conceptualized as a hybrid of evaluation (discussed below) and feedback. Mid-rotation structured feedback allows the student to "change course" before the experience has ended. At the end of the experience, the teacher may summarize the learner's performance for the final evauation and outline "next steps" for the learner to take to their next experience. Formal feedback may take from five to twenty minutes.

## ❖ Why Is Feedback So Hard to Do?

Many of us find it hard to give critical feedback. One reason is the conflict between our different roles. We see ourselves as advocates helping trainees succeed but at the same time recognize our roles as a protector of society by ensuring good patient care and as a physician maintaining the standards of the profession. With these divided loyalties, we may be hesitant to give critical feedback, fearing loss of our advocacy role. Another reason we find feedback so difficult is that it is time consuming to plan, execute, and document feedback sessions. Finally, we also may be uncertain of how to do it, due to lack of personal experience and instruction.

## ❖ Feedback Tips

The following paragraphs explain how to go about providing feedback that is respectful of the learner, time-efficient, and most likely to result in the desired change in learner behavior (see Summary of Feedback Tips in Appendix B on page 164).

*Set Expectations*
Feedback that is expected is more easily accepted by the learner. Set the expectation from the beginning that feedback will be given regularly and its purpose is continuous improvement. Give both scheduled and incident-related feedback and identify clearly that what you are doing is providing feedback.

> **Good example of setting expectations:** "I will be giving you feedback most every day on your performance and we'll meet in the middle of the rotation and at its end to discuss your progress."
>
> **Poor example of setting expectations:** "I think we better talk since you don't seem to be doing very well."

*Give Feedback That Is Timely and Specific*
Learners get the most from feedback when it is timely (given as close to the incident event as possible) and when it is specific. By giving specific examples, the learner has a better chance of repeating the desired behaviors (catching the learner doing something well) and not repeating undesirable behavior. When giving feedback, explain the consequence of the behavior to reinforce the message.

**Good example of timely and specific feedback:** "I liked how you repeated the patient's question back to him. This shows you are listening and interested."

**Poor example of timely and specific feedback:** "I meant to tell you last week that you did a poor job communicating follow-up instructions to my patients."

*Give Limited Feedback*

Keep your feedback agenda limited, focusing on the points that are most important to hear. Don't overwhelm the learner with too much information but rather provide manageable chunks of information that the learner can act on.

**Good example of limiting feedback:** "I can see that you have never started a patient on insulin before. Read about initiating insulin therapy in patients with type 2 diabetes and we can discuss this patient again in the morning."

**Poor example of limiting feedback:** You seem to know nothing about caring for patients with diabetes, including when to initiate insulin therapy, how to monitor therapy, therapeutic goals or how to follow up on treatment. You also lack confidence when talking with patients and give confusing instructions, and your notes are disorganized."

*Focus the Feedback on Describing Behaviors*

It is easier for learners to hear non-judgmental, descriptive feedback. Express your feedback in terms of behaviors that the learner can change without attacking the learner's self-esteem. It is perfectly acceptable to express your feelings about a learner's performance such as, "I was excited (disappointed, confused) that you…" provided that you also affirm your belief that the learner has ability to change and wants to do better.

**Good example of non-judgmental feedback:** "I am not sure the patient understood your instructions. Let's discuss ways you can improve your communication skills."

**Poor example of non-judgmental feedback:** "You are aloof and uncaring and cannot be bothered to communicate even simple instructions."

### Focus Feedback on Behavior That Can Change

Focus your feedback on behaviors that the learner can control. Feedback that learners cannot act on is pointless and frustrating.

**Good example of feedback that can change behavior:** "Patients sometimes have trouble understanding you. I recommend that you speak more slowly and frequently check to see if you are being understood."

**Poor example of feedback that can change behavior:** "Your accent is so pronounced that no one can understand you."

### Direct Feedback Towards Future Behavior

Help the learner reflect on and analyze what went right and what went wrong within the context of how they can change future performance. Focus on decisions and actions the learner can take.

**Good example of future directed feedback:** "Next time if you have trouble finding the correct dose of a drug, come and get me out of the examination room and we will find it together."

**Poor example of future directed feedback:** "You are lucky I caught that dosing error. Don't let this happen again."

### Use Self-Assessment as Part of Feedback

Many experts advocate beginning feedback by asking the learner for their self-assessment (7). You might ask, "What went well and what could you have done better?" Typically, the learner will bring up the same points you wish to discuss, allowing you to reinforce them. If the learner brings up issues not on your list, you can address them before moving on to your agenda.

In more formal feedback sessions, learners can perform a self-assessment by filling out a copy of the institution's evaluation form. This self-assessment exercise provides information on the learner's insight and is an excellent opportunity to begin a discussion with the learner about his or her performance. Overall, the use of self-assessment promotes an interactive dialog between you and the learner and removes from you some of the onus of evaluation.

*Use the "Feedback Sandwich"*

Many educators use some variation of the "feedback sandwich" for both formal and brief feedback and studies have verified its usefulness (8). The "feedback sandwich" has three components delivered in the following order:

- What was done right
- What was done wrong
- What to do next time

When you begin, it is wise to ask the learner's permission, "I need to give you some feedback, is this a good time?" Initiate the conversation with a positive comment so the learner will be more receptive to the subsequent "meat" of the feedback sandwich, the things the learner did not do well and needs to improve. Alternatively, you can begin by asking the learner for their self-assessment ("What went well and what could you have done better?") and all you need to do is verify the learner's assessment and provide specific examples of the identified behaviors. Limit the amount of feedback by focusing on the points that are most important. Whenever possible, link feedback to the learning objectives provided by the sponsoring institution or to the Learner Contract (see When the Learner Arrives in Chapter 3 on page 28). Finally, cap the feedback "sandwich" with detailed instructions for improvement and suggest opportunities to practice. Remember to follow up with positive feedback and praise if the learner is able to "get it right." Box 8-1 contains examples of short, relevant feedback.

The risk of the feedback sandwich is that the learner becomes conditioned to a positive comment as something that precedes a corrective one. Therefore it is helpful to occasionally rearrange the sandwich. It is also helpful, when possible, to dampen the sting of the criticism with an acknowledgment that you have made that same mistake or that making

## Box 8-1. Relevant Feedback "Sandwiches"

► "I like the way you examined the heart. You were methodical, going through each step of inspection, palpation, percussion, and auscultation. However, I noticed that you used only the diaphragm of the stethoscope and not the bell. The bell is important when listening for low-pitched sounds. On subsequent patients, I want you to listen with the bell at each major area. This will allow you to better hear the low-pitched sounds."

► "Patients seem to like you. Yet, some patients seem to be frustrated when you don't give them enough time to answer your questions. Be patient. Wait several seconds, check to see if they have anything they would like to add, and then move on. This will save you time in the long run."

mistakes is part of the process of learning. Feedback is offered without hesitation and contains the facts about what was wrong, what should have been done, and why. Hesitancy when offering feedback can be perceived by the learner as a sign that what happened is too upsetting to say. After your message is conveyed, ask the learner for their comments. You can add a final comment that affirms your confidence that the learner is capable of changing and that you will help them.

To summarize, feedback is more effective with a little advanced planning. Inform the learner at the beginning of the rotation that feedback will be provided throughout the experience. Select an appropriate time and place and provide it privately as soon as possible after the learning event. Select only one or two important items to discuss, and keep the discussion to approximately five minutes or less. Serve your version of the "feedback sandwich," be sure that the learner understands what has been said, and arrange for a follow-up.

❖ **Time-Saving Tips for Giving Feedback**

- Effective feedback does not have to be verbal. Preprinted feed-back notes with the notation "Well done" or "Needs improvement" and specific notation of the observed behavior is found by students to be more constructive, timely, and concrete than verbal feedback (9). See an example of a feedback note form in Appendix A on page 141.
- When observing learners, keep a pocket card with notes (including "catching them doing something well") to help you remember specifics for later. Alternatively, keep copies of your feedback notes to learners (above) to remind you of past performance.
- If a learner is with you for several weeks, try focusing feedback on one specific skill area each week, e.g., one week focus on communication, another week focus on physical examination. This enables you to be more efficient by concentrating on only one specific learning goal (which may be chosen by the learner).

❖ **Barriers to Effective Feedback**

While men and women learners equally value constructive feedback, studies show that men and women do not receive feedback in equal amounts or with similar content (10). Women preceptors are more likely to give feedback on clinical skills to male learners than to female learners. The learner-preceptor combination associated with giving the most feedback is male preceptor and learner; the worst is female preceptor and learner. Women preceptors are more likely to comment positively on male learner's maturity and/or character and negatively on female learner's clinical skills. It is important for preceptors to acknowledge the possibility of gender bias in giving feedback and guard against it.

Often, learners don't recognize or remember feedback (11). This can be overcome by prefacing feedback with the statement, "Let me give you some feedback." Other common barriers to effective feedback is the fear that it may upset learners, but provided that feedback, even negative feedback, is given privately, these fears have not been realized. Some preceptors give feedback but soften the criticism to a degree that the message is lost. Given an opportunity to plan for and provide written feedback, these same preceptors provide more critical feedback as compared to the face-to-face encounter (12). Consider planning and rehearsing your feedback before meeting with the learner or using written feedback notes. See Table 8-1 for information on barriers to effective feedback.

## Table 8-1. Barriers to Effective Feedback

| Barrier | Impact | Potential Approach |
|---|---|---|
| Worried about upsetting learner with feedback | Feedback is not provided, or infrequently provided | Dismiss these fears; learners crave and value feedback and associate it with high quality teaching. |
| Learners don't recall getting feedback or remember feedback content | Learners are dissatisfied with learning environment or fail to act on feedback | Label feedback prior to its delivery with, "Let me give you some feedback." |
| Gender bias | Men and women learners receive different amounts of feedback and of different content | Be sensitive to the possibility of gender differences when giving feedback. |
| Feedback "too soft", does not contain needed critical component | Learners do not improve skills and persist with undesirable behaviors | Consider planning and rehearsing feedback ahead of delivery or giving written feedback notes. |
| Feedback too general (for example, "You can do better") | Learners cannot improve and become frustrated | Develop a system of recording specific skills that need to improve or behaviors that need to change. Use the notes to provide the learner with detailed examples and suggestions for improvement. |

## ❖ What Is the Difference Between Feedback and Evaluation?

It is sometimes difficult to understand the difference between feedback and evaluation. Evaluation assigns a numerical or descriptive "value" to the learner's performance (see Summary of Evaluation in Appendix B on page

165). The value placed on the learner's performance typically is judged against goals established for the learning experience. In a real sense, evaluation occurs throughout the educational experience. It is in the assessment (observing) and evaluation (assigning value) process that allows you generate and provide feedback to the learner. Under ideal circumstances, assessment, evaluation, and feedback all take place during and after each learner-patient encounter but realistically it happens as time permits. As such, most preceptors equate evaluation with assigning a grade at the end of the rotation. In keeping with this concept, this section addresses aspects of the final (or summative) end-of-rotation evaluation.

### ❖ Why Is Summative Evaluation Important?

Typically, medical schools and residency programs collect summative evaluations from preceptors and faculty to meet the following educational needs:

- Determining learner competence and identifying learner strengths and weaknesses
- Identifying strengths and weaknesses of the curriculum
- Making decisions about retention and promotion
- Providing information to outside institutions (e.g., for internship applications)
- Maintaining accreditation of the institution
- Providing legal documentation

### ❖ Basic Steps in the Evaluation Process

Most training programs provide a set of learning goals and objectives or competencies that should be reviewed with the learner at the beginning of the office experience. Most institutions list desired knowledge, attitudinal, and skill competencies (analytic model) on the evaluation form. An example is the Core Medicine Clerkship Curriculum Guide of the training problems and core competencies for students enrolled in the basic internal medicine clerkship (www.im.org/CDIM/CurriculumGuide/OnlineCDIMCurriculum.pdf). An evaluation rating scale measures the degree to which the learner mastered the learning goals and objectives.

It is a good idea to review the evaluation with the learner at the beginning of the experience, giving him or her advanced notice of what will be evaluated (see When the Learner Arrives in Chapter 3 on page 28). The evaluation form is a succinct document which in part functions to "communicate" the basic goals of the experience. To fill out the form accurately, you must have a sound and efficient method of collecting performance data, including information derived from some or all of the following sources:

- Direct observation of learner performance
- Written records (e.g., progress notes, histories, physical examination findings)
- Oral patient presentations
- Responses to probing, hypothetical, and alternative scenario questions
- "Homework" assignments
- Interactions with office staff
- Patient comments or measures of satisfaction
- Learner self-evaluation

The most reliable method of collecting performance data is direct observation, e.g., watching the learner take a history, perform an examination, or counsel a patient. Do not "infer" performance in the history and physical examination based upon indirect sources such as case presentations and the written record because these sources of information are likely to inflate the learner's abilities (13). Rather than observing a learner-patient interaction from beginning to end, it may be more efficient to observe the learner performing parts of the history or examination on different patients over time (see The One-Minute Observation in Chapter 5 on page 63 and Summary of the One-Minute Observation in Appendix B on page 158). For example, over several days, you may observe the learner taking a focused history on one patient, performing a cardiovascular examination on a second patient, and counseling a third. The American Board of Internal Medicine has developed the "mini Clinical Evaluation Exercise (mini-CEX)" form, which is a useful tool to record short patient encounters and help organize your feedback (see page 143 in Appendix A).

Using simple methods, you can assess the learner's ability to synthesize and present patient data in a concise and helpful manner. The learner's knowledge and judgment can be evaluated by using the teaching Microskills or other learner-centered precepting models (see Chapter 5). The process of having the student make a commitment, followed by probing for supporting information, is an efficient evaluation and teaching technique. By using hypothetical and alternative questioning techniques (see Box 8-2), you can assess depth of knowledge. The learner's progress notes can be reviewed for clarity, organization, accuracy, and understanding regarding the assessment and plan.

Observing how the learner interacts with other members of the office staff and soliciting their comments can provide other sources of important evaluation data. Patients are another good source of primary data, and their comments can be collected formally by asking them to fill out a written survey (see Patient Satisfaction Form in Appendix A on page 144) or informally by asking them some casual questions (14,15). Patient feedback is a powerful motivating factor for modifying learner behavior (6).

Learners should be expected to follow up on reading assignments with their compliance and thoroughness reflected in the evaluation.

---

### Box 8-2. Questioning Techniques

**Use of a Hypothetical Question**

▶ "I agree that three days of sulfamethoxazole-trimethoprim is an appropriate choice for this young woman with cystitis. How would you modify your treatment if she were diabetic with a fever and flank pain?"

**Use of an Alternative Question**

▶ "What might be the expected outcome if we treated her cystitis with ampicillin rather than sulfamethoxazole-trimethoprim?"

If you have concerns about a learner's knowledge base, skills, or professionalism, contact the program early in the process! Program and clerkship directors can tell you if this is a new or recurring problem, help you resolve the issue, or at least help you and the learner deal with the possibility of a bad evaluation.

## ❖ What Are Common Types of Evaluation Errors?

Physicians who evaluate learners are prone to make one or more rating errors. Some of the errors are understandable given the natural reluctance to submit a poor evaluation that may adversely affect promotion or retention in the training program. Other errors reflect a poor understanding of the evaluation system and its role in identifying sub-optimal performance at a time when remediation is most effective. Common rating errors include:

- The "halo/horn" effect
- Restriction of range
- Evaluating nonperformance attributes
- The Lake Wobegon effect

*The "Halo/Horn" Effect*

The "halo/horn" effect is evaluation biased by the learner's past ratings rather than on objective evaluation of current performance. For example, having heard that a learner is an outstanding student, you submit an "excellent" evaluation despite an "average" actual performance in your office: "Dr. Smith said the student was terrific; maybe my expectations for the student are just too high." Conversely you have a good experience with a resident but think, "The other preceptors say that he is a terrible resident; maybe I should give him a lower grade."

Susceptibility to the halo/horn effect is commonly the result of preceptor inexperience or a lack of confidence. It is always best to make your evaluation based on your observations and trust your instincts. Document your decisions and, whenever possible, support them with specific examples of behaviors that help justify your evaluation rating.

*Restriction of Range*

Restriction of range refers to the tendency to circle the same numerical rating for all competencies, rather than fully considering and rating each characteristic separately. For example, on a five-point scale representing performance attributes from "unsatisfactory" to "superior," the preceptor circles the same score for all the characteristics being evaluated. Although efficient for the preceptor, this rating strategy increases the chances of submitting an inaccurate evaluation.

*Rating Nonperformance Attributes*

Factoring in "nonperformance attributes" when evaluating a competency is another source of error. For example, "laziness" in a bright student who has mastered the cognitive competencies should be reflected in the attitudinal competency section, not the cognitive section of the evaluation. Precisely identifying the categories of poor performance has important implications for learner remediation. Obviously, a remediation program focused on enhancing content knowledge would be wasted on a learner whose attitude needs improvement. Conversely, a nice, eager student with poor physical examination and oral presentation skills may be given a higher rating than deserved because "he's such a nice student."

*The Lake Wobegon Effect*

This common error entails rating all students "above average" and fails to discriminate between the inadequate student, the student meeting all expectations, and the truly exceptional student. The poorly performing student is not properly identified and fails to receive corrective remediation. In the long run, the Lake Wobegon effect can erode student and institution trust in you as an evaluator and as an effective faculty person. Discipline yourself to use the entire range of the evaluation tool and justify the evaluation with specific observed behaviors, skills, attitudes, and written work. Conversely, if using a numeric scale, it is important to know what your institution's "average" is so as to not penalize good learners if "grade inflation" is an issue at your institution.

## ❖ Evaluation Using the GRADE Strategy

Many of the evaluation errors can be avoided by preparing throughout the clinical experience for the final face-to-face evaluation encounter. By integrating preparation into the ongoing clinical experience, the process becomes much easier and more reliable. A useful mnemonic, GRADE has been proposed by Langlois and co-workers to outline the necessary steps for a more satisfactory and effective evaluation process (see Table 8-2) (16). See page 167 in Appendix B for a summary of the GRADE evaluation strategy.

## Table 8-2. The GRADE Strategy for Evaluation

**G** - Get Ready (see "Before the Learner Arrives," page 25 [Chapter 3])

    Review course expectations and the evaluation form

    Articulate your expectations for the learner

    Schedule the end of experience evaluation meeting

**R** - Review expectations with the learner (see "Before the Learner Arrives," Page 25 [Chapter 3])

    Meet with the learner early in the experience

    Determine the learners knowledge and skill level (see "Summary of the Learning Experience," page 154 [Appendix B, Summaries and Checklists for Preceptors]

    Review the program's goals, your goals, and the learner's goals

    Describe the evaluation process

**A** - Assess (see Chapter 7, Learner Feedback and Evaluation)

    Observe

    Record

    Provide feedback regularly

    Have learner self-assess

**D** - Discuss assessment (see Chapter 7, Learner Feedback and Evaluation)

    Formal meeting

    Learner and preceptor fill out evaluation forms

    Compare evaluations together

    Discuss differences and whether expectations were met

**E** - End with a grade (see Chapter 7, Learner Feedback and Evaluation)

    Complete evaluation form

    Support your evaluation with examples

Modified with permission: Langlois JP, Thach S. Evaluation using the GRADE strategy. Fam Med. 2001;33:158-60.

## ❖ The RIME Evaluation Framework

Pangaro's developmental model for performance expectations and feedback (17) integrates learner achievement, provides a framework for putting learner problems in perspective, and is highly intuitive, making it easy to articulate and apply (see Summary of the RIME Evaluation Framework in Appendix B on page 166). RIME is a mnemonic for the progressively complex and sophisticated clinical skills shown in Box 8-3.

The RIME model differs from other evaluation models in that it is "synthetic." "Analytic" evaluation models ask you to evaluate attainment of knowledge, attitude, and skills separately. Unfortunately, most preceptors do not conceptualize learner performance according to these attributes. Outside the milieu of full-time educators, these concepts are somewhat foreign, and the format is not intuitive. The RIME evaluation framework avoids the somewhat artificial distinction of evaluating the individual components of medical competencies and uses a "developmental" approach instead. Each step in the RIME model represents a synthesis of knowledge,

---

### Box 8-3. RIME Evaluation Framework

**Reporter**
  - ▶ Consistently collects and reports data in an accurate, organized way.

**Interpreter**
  - ▶ Consistently interprets history clues, physical-examination findings, and laboratory results; creates and prioritizes problem lists and creates and justifies a differential diagnosis.

**Manager**
  - ▶ Consistently selects and applies appropriate diagnostic and treatment options that best meets the patient's needs.

**Educator**
  - ▶ Identifies and addresses knowledge gaps using evidence based approaches and educates the patient and colleagues using their knowledge, clinical reasoning, and analytic skills.

attitude, and skill that is practiced and mastered as a learner progresses from the preclinical years of medical school through residency training, and transitions from a novice to an expert clinician. Mastering each level depends on mastering the previous level.

RIME is also useful because it is a much more reliable way to evaluate a learner's skills. Different teachers who have been trained to use the RIME evaluation framework can "reliably" evaluate learners' skills (the ability to get the same results as other raters). The RIME framework also has strong predictive validity characteristics; in other words, the results predict measures of future performance, such as on the end of clerkship examination and in an internship (18,19). The RIME framework has also been used to evaluate learners' professionalism (20). However, for all its shortcomings, you will probably be given an analytic evaluation form asking you to rate various knowledge, attitude, and skill attributes with a numerical scale. In this situation, the RIME model is so simple and intuitive that you can use it to help guide your personal evaluation of the learner and then translate the results of your RIME evaluation to whatever format the sponsoring institution requires.

### What Skills Should a "Reporter" Have?

A "reporter" is mastering data collection and reporting. Learners who have mastered reporting can efficiently and accurately collect history and physical-examination data, can recognize normal and abnormal findings, and can identify and label new problems. Additionally, they are capable of communicating this information orally and in writing in an organized way. Mastery of skills at the reporter level is expected of all third-year students.

### What Skills Should an "Interpreter" Have Mastered?

Mastery of interpreter skills means that the learner interprets data, develops a differential diagnosis, prioritizes problems and differential diagnoses from most likely to least likely, and follows up on and interprets results of physical findings and diagnostic tests. Acquisition of this skill level marks the transition from "bystander" to active participant in patient care. Mastery of this skill level is associated with a high passing or honors grade for a third-year student and is expected of senior students and interns (first-year residents).

*What Skills Define Mastery at "Manager" Level?*
Managers determine when action is necessary (versus "watchful waiting"), select the best diagnostic and therapeutic options, and customize care according to patient circumstances and preferences. They take the initiative to search out answers and alternatives to clinical questions. Mastery at the manager level requires advanced knowledge, confidence, clinical reasoning and judgment, and is most often attained by junior and senior (second- and third-year) residents and practitioners.

*What Is an "Educator"?*
An "Educator" identifies knowledge gaps and takes the initiative to address these gaps. Educators synthesize and share new knowledge with others and understand the uses and limitations of evidence in the care of patients. These skills take drive, insight, and maturity, and are most likely to be present in senior residents and practitioners. See page 145 in Appendix A for an example of a behaviorally anchored RIME evaluation framework with explicit descriptions of three different performance levels: Areas for Improvement, Competent, and Strength.

## ❖ Using the RIME Model to Assess Case Presentations

When assessing a learner's case presentation, you can ask yourself where the learner is located on the RIME scale (21). Is the learner at correct developmental level and should this learner be praised or coached to improve skills. If used properly, the RIME framework should suggest specific areas of improvement. See Table 8-3 for an example of using the RIME model to assess a case presentation and coach the learner.

## Table 8-3. RIME Evaluation of Case Presentations

| RIME Level | Case Presentation | Assessment and Coaching |
|---|---|---|
| Reporter | The patient is a 57-year-old man with 3-month history of pain in the left calf when he walks 2 blocks. The pain is relieved with rest but returns with walking. He smokes cigarettes and also has hypertension treated with atenolol and lisinopril. His blood pressure is 142/86 mm Hg. Pulses are decreased in the left foot, but normal in the groin. [Learner ends presentation ends here.] | Excellent presentation. Above average for a third-year student, expected performance for an experienced 4th-year student or first-year resident. Coach the learner to "interpret" the findings by making a commitment to a diagnosis or differential diagnosis. |
| Interpreter | I believe the patient has peripheral artery disease because of the constant association of pain with exertion and relief with rest, history of smoking, and hypertension. I think spinal stenosis is less likely because of his age. [Learner ends presentation here.] | Learner is able to synthesize the data from the history and physical examination and can support a correct but limited differential diagnosis. Some 4th-year students and most first-year residents should be at this level. Coach the learner to commit to a management plan. |
| Manager | We can confirm the diagnosis by measuring the ankle-brachial index [Learner ends presentation here]. | Learner recognizes a simple, non-invasive office-based test that can confirm the diagnosis and grade the severity but neglected to address the smoking and blood pressure. This level is expected of most first-year residents and higher. Coach the learner to consider all elements that may have a bearing on the case. |
| Educator | Guidelines from the Seventh Report of the Joint National Committee on Prevention, Detection, Evaluation and Treatment of High Blood Pressure recommend aggressive blood pressure control in patient with peripheral artery disease to < 130/80 mm Hg. Although the beta-blocker may worsen his symptoms of claudication, it may be offset by increased protection from coronary artery disease; but I don't know for sure and I need to look this up. He needs a clear, unambiguous message to stop smoking and we need to find out if he is interested in stopping as smoking cessation is associated with a reduction in all-cause mortality. | Learner demonstrates past learning, willingness to share knowledge and recognizes own deficiencies with a plan to address them. This level is expected of senior residents and practicing physicians. The coaching task is to clearly commend the learner's grasp of the content and reinforce the necessity to identify knowledge gaps and how to address them. |

## ❖ When and How Should the Evaluation Session Be Scheduled?

In contrast to feedback, a summative evaluation (as we have defined it) occurs once at the end of the teaching experience. A time should be set aside to review the evaluation with the learner before the evaluation form is returned to the sponsoring institution. Having the learner fill out a copy of the evaluation before this meeting can be a helpful transition into the evaluation discussion. This sets the stage for the upcoming discussion by reminding the learner of the learning goals and evaluation criteria. Letting the learner summarize his or her self-assessment using the evaluation form also can provide a comfortable transition to your own observations. Additionally, self-evaluation provides an opportunity to practice the type of "reflective practice" professional behavior expected of physicians in the "real world" (7).

After the learner has summarized his or her performance, you can confirm, elaborate, or modify the self-assessment with your own observations and conclusions. You will be surprised how accurately learners evaluate their own performance, particularly in areas of needed improvement. The rare learner who fails to identify important areas of improvement may have poor insight, and this should be brought to his or her (and the institution's) attention.

As with feedback, you need to be as specific as possible in the evaluation process, citing examples of behaviors that support your evaluation decisions. It is helpful to have the learner sign the evaluation report at the end of the session, indicating that it was reviewed with him or her.

Fill out the institution's evaluation form as soon as you can. The longer you wait, the more difficult it becomes to remember the specifics of the learner's performance. In this case, you might have a good feeling for the overall performance of the learner but will be unable to justify your conclusions. Make a copy of the evaluation form and file it. This ensures against the evaluation being lost at the sponsoring institution and having to fill out another form. Finally, return the evaluation on time to the course director.

# REFERENCES

1. **Heidenreich C, Lye P, Simpson D, Lourich M.** The search for effective and efficient ambulatory teaching methods through the literature. Pediatrics. 2000;105:231-7.
2. **Skeff KM.** Enhancing teaching effectiveness and vitality in the ambulatory setting. J Gen Intern Med. 1988;3(Suppl):S26-33.
3. **McGee SR, Irby DM.** Teaching in the outpatient clinic: practical tips. J Gen Intern Med. 1997;12(Suppl):S34-40.
4. **Ende J.** Feedback in clinical medical education. JAMA. 1983;250:777-81.
5. **Schultz KW, Kirby J, Delva D, et al.** Medical Students' and Residents' preferred site characteristics and preceptor behaviours for learning in the ambulatory setting: a cross-sectional survey. BMC Med Educ. 2004;4:12.
6. **Cope DW, Linn LS, Leake BD, Barrett PA.** Modification of residents' behavior by preceptor feedback of patient satisfaction. J Gen Intern Med. 1986;1:394-8.
7. **Branch WT Jr, Paranjape A.** Feedback and reflection: teaching methods for clinical settings. Acad Med. 2002;77:1185-8.
8. **Anderson WA, Malacrea RF.** Giving Constructive Feedback: A Professional Development Workshop Package. East Lansing, MI: Office of Medical Education Research and Development, College of Human Medicine, Michigan State University; 1987.
9. **Schum TR, Krippendorf RL, Biernat KA.** Simple feedback notes enhance specificity of feedback to learners. Ambul Pediatr. 2003;3:9-11.
10. **Carney PA, Dietrich AJ, Eliassen S, et al.** Differences in ambulatory teaching and learning by gender match of preceptors and students. Fam Med. 2000;32:618-23.
11. **Sostok MA, Coberly L, Rouan G.** Feedback process between faculty and students. Acad Med. 2002;77:267.
12. **Colletti LM.** Difficulty with negative feedback: face-to-face evaluation of junior medical student clinical performance results in grade inflation. J Surg Res. 2000;90:82-7.
13. **Pulito AR, Donnelly MB, Plymale M, Mentzer RM Jr.** What do faculty observe of medical students' clinical performance? Teach Learn Med. 2006;18:99-104.
14. **Weaver MJ, Ow CL, Walker DJ, Degenhardt EF.** A questionnaire for patients' evaluations of their physicians' humanistic behaviors. J Gen Intern Med. 1993;8:135-9.
15. **Tamblyn R, Benaroya S, Snell L, et al.** The feasibility and value of using patient satisfaction ratings to evaluate internal medicine residents. J Gen Intern Med. 1994;9:149-52.
16. **Langlois JP, Thach S.** Evaluation using the GRADE strategy. Fam Med. 2001;33:158-60.
17. **Pangaro L.** A new vocabulary and other innovations for improving descriptive in-training evaluations. Acad Med. 1999;74:41-5.
18. **Hemmer PA, Pangaro L.** The effectiveness of formal evaluation sessions during clinical clerkships in better identifying students with marginal funds of knowledge. Acad Med. 1997;72:641-3.
19. **Lavin B, Pangaro L.** Internship ratings as a validity outcome measure for an evaluation system to identify inadequate clerkship performance. Acad Med. 1998;73:998-1002.
20. **Hemmer PA, Hawkins R, Jackson JL, Pangaro LN.** Assessing how well three evaluation methods detect deficiencies in medical students' professionalism in two settings of an internal medicine clerkship. Acad Med. 2000;75:167-73.
21. **Sepdham D, Julka M, Hofmann L, Dobbie A.** Using the RIME model for learner assessment and feedback. Fam Med. 2007;39:161-3.

# 9

# Preceptor Evaluation and Teaching Improvement

## ❖ How Will You Be Evaluated?

Preceptor evaluations by learners allow the sponsoring institution to monitor the quality of the educational program and to make improvements where they are needed. Most often, preceptors are evaluated by students or residents at the end of the rotation using a standard evaluation form (see Preceptor Evaluation Form in Appendix B on page 168). Although many programs attempt to get the learner to complete the preceptor's evaluation before receiving their end-of-rotation evaluation, this does not always occur. The evaluation form reflects the learning goals of the experience and asks to what extent you were able to help the learner achieve those goals. This process is identical to that used for full-time faculty at medical schools and residency programs, yet it is not always comfortable. Make it a practice to solicit feedback from your learners throughout the rotation. Soliciting feedback repeatedly from the trainee will allow you to adjust your teaching along the way and prevent being surprised with critical evaluations at the end.

At some point, a summary of all your learners' evaluations will be returned to you. This often takes place after a large number of learners have rotated through your office to increase the sample size and relia-

bility of the process. Some delay in receiving the evaluations is often delib-
erate to ensure the anonymity of the learners completing the evaluations.
Most institutions will summarize the scores of the learners and provide a
mean score for each category on the evaluation form. If the institution's
program is large enough, it will also provide comparison data consisting of
a mean score derived from all other preceptor evaluations. This will allow
you to compare your performance against your peers. Written comments
from the learners usually are collected for your review. Usually the authors
of the comments are not identified.

Despite the fact you have sacrificed time and, sometimes, income to be
a preceptor, your evaluations may not always reflect your efforts. It is
important to be philosophical about the evaluations and to recognize that
you will never be able to please everyone; however, the evaluations can provide you with important information, and good teachers, like good doctors,
do best when they practice "reflective teaching" with continuous improvement in mind.


## ❖ How Can You Improve Your Teaching?

In the context of professional practice, reflection is essential in the educational experiences of both learners and teachers. Reflection has been
defined as a "thought, idea, or opinion formed as the result of mediation."
Medical educators supplement this definition to include consideration of
the larger context, the meaning, and the implications of an experience or
action (1). You must be able to reflect on your instruction if you are to
identify ways of improving it (2,3).

Reflection during the teaching process involves making necessary
adjustments to each changing teaching situation. For example, if your
evaluation says, "the preceptor doesn't give enough general information
(teaches too much specialty information)," you might be more specific
about referring the learner to resources or even browse the student syllabus to more accurately teach to the expected level. Inflexibility on your
part at this stage can result in poor teaching performance. An example of
inflexibility is continuing to explain the reasons for selecting one therapy

over another when it is obvious that the learner is unclear about the basic disease process. The preceptor who can, through reflection, recognize a learner's difficulty, drop the discussion of therapy, and substitute one about disease mechanism and natural history is more likely to be successful.

For many preceptors, reflection after teaching provides the impetus for change and improvement. Assessing what went well and what went wrong are key steps in this self-evaluation process. Excellent preceptors use this information to make their teaching more effective and relevant for the learner. Less effective teachers never change or even consider the need to change.

Teaching failures will occur; they are an integral part of the process. However, when confronted with failure, there are several things you can do. First, be realistic; even the best of teachers have bad days when nothing seems to work. Second, keep your "antennae" out to recognize the parts that were and were not successful. If you are lucky, you can ask for and receive useful feedback; however, this may not occur, so you must personally observe what engages the learner and adjust your teaching accordingly (3).

## ❖ Workshops, Courses, Peer Site Visits, and Additional Resources

As the need for community-based preceptors increases, so does the awareness for faculty development to improve teaching skills. Not surprisingly, community-based preceptors have had less formal skills training than their academic colleagues. Compared to full-time faculty, community-based preceptors identify giving feedback and evaluation of learners as their most significant general teaching skills deficits (4). When asked about specific topics, community preceptors identify time management (while teaching) as the most important topic, followed by teaching evidence-based medicine skills (4).

Faculty-development courses are usually scheduled over a two- or three-day period, but many formats can be designed to accommodate community physicians. Perceptions of these courses are typically positive, and the benefit of attending often exceeds the participants' expectations: they report improvement in their ability to foster a constructive learning climate, to communicate goals, to provide feedback, and to teach overall (5).

Peer site visits also improve teaching. Participants in such visits indicate that these provide a unique and helpful opportunity for reflective discussion. When direct observation of faculty teaching is combined with written feedback, faculty improve their learner-centered teaching and use of the microskills teaching model (6). Others see site visits as opportunities to validate and affirm their approaches to teaching and to foster a strong sense of collegiality (7).

Selected faculty development resources are listed in Appendix C, Resources for Preceptors and additional independent learning resources to improve teaching skills can be found on the electronic enhancement to Teaching in Your Office "Selected Faculty Development Materials" at www.acponline.org/acp_press/teaching_in_your_office.

## REFERENCES

1. **Branch WT Jr, Paranjape A.** Feedback and reflection: teaching methods for clinical settings. Acad Med. 2002;77:1185-8.
2. **Skeff KM, Bowen JL, Irby DM.** Protecting time for teaching in the ambulatory care setting. Acad Med. 1997;72:694-7.
3. **Pinsky LE, Irby DM.** "If at first you don't succeed": using failure to improve teaching. Acad Med. 1997;72:973-6.
4. **Houston TK, Ferenchick GS, Clark JM, et al.** Faculty development needs. J Gen Intern Med. 2004;19:375-9.
5. **Skeff KM, Stratos GA, Bergen MR, et al.** Regional teaching improvement programs for community-based teachers. Am J Med. 1999;106:76-80.
6. **Regan-Smith M, Hirschmann K, Iobst W.** Direct observation of faculty with feedback: an effective means of improving patient-centered and learner-centered teaching skills. Teach Learn Med. 2007;19:278-86.
7. **Bing-You RG, Renfrew RA, Hampton SH.** Faculty development of community-based preceptors through a collegial site-visit program. Teach Learn Med. 1999;11:100-4.

# APPENDIX A

## Tools for Preceptors

## ❖ Clinical Skills Inventory

*To be filled out by the learner at or before the orientation.*
*See "When the Learner Arrives" on page 28.*

**Student Name** _____

*Part I.* ***To help your preceptor improve your clinical skills, please indicate your experience by checking the appropriate box.***

| Physical Examination | No Experience | Some Experience | Much Experience |
| --- | --- | --- | --- |
| 1. Adolescent | ❑ | ❑ | ❑ |
| 2. Complete adult | ❑ | ❑ | ❑ |
| 3. System focused | ❑ | ❑ | ❑ |
| 4. Breast | ❑ | ❑ | ❑ |
| 5. Pelvic | ❑ | ❑ | ❑ |
| 6. Rectal | ❑ | ❑ | ❑ |
| 7. Prostate | ❑ | ❑ | ❑ |
| 8. Cardiovascular | ❑ | ❑ | ❑ |
| 9. Abdominal | ❑ | ❑ | ❑ |
| 10. Pulmonary | ❑ | ❑ | ❑ |
| 11. Musculoskeletal | ❑ | ❑ | ❑ |

## Part II. *Are there other areas in which you feel that you need specific instruction? Please check the appropriate boxes.*

| Procedures | No Experience | Some Experience | Much Experience |
|---|---|---|---|
| 1. Electrocardiogram interpretation | ❏ | ❏ | ❏ |
| 2. Flexible sigmoidoscopy | ❏ | ❏ | ❏ |
| 3. Gram stain interpretation | ❏ | ❏ | ❏ |
| 4. Joint aspiration/injection | ❏ | ❏ | ❏ |
| 5. KOH (skin) | ❏ | ❏ | ❏ |
| 6. Soft-tissue trigger injection | ❏ | ❏ | ❏ |
| 7. Pap smear | ❏ | ❏ | ❏ |
| 8. Testing stool for blood | ❏ | ❏ | ❏ |
| 9. Throat culture | ❏ | ❏ | ❏ |
| 10. Urinalysis (dip stick) | ❏ | ❏ | ❏ |
| 11. Urinalysis (microscopic) | ❏ | ❏ | ❏ |
| 12. Wet mount/vaginal | ❏ | ❏ | ❏ |
| 13. Skin biopsy | ❏ | ❏ | ❏ |

## Part III. *Are there other areas in which you feel that you need specific instruction?*

_____
_____
_____
_____
_____

## ❖ Learner Contract

*To be given to the learner at the time of orientation.*
*See "When the Learner Arrives" on page 28.*

**Student Name** _____

**Preceptor Name** _____

### Part I.  Student's Goals
**List the three most important goals you have for this preceptorship.**

1. _____
2. _____
3. _____

**List specific strategies you suggest for accomplishing these goals.**

_____
_____
_____
_____

### Part II.  Preceptor's Goals
**List the three most important areas on which you believe the student should focus:**

1. _____
2. _____
3. _____

**List strategies you suggest for addressing these areas:**

_____

_____

_____

_____

## Part III.  Summary
**Performance goals and expectations are:**

_____

_____

_____

_____

**Student Name** _____ **Date** _____

**Preceptor Name** _____ **Date** _____

## ❖ Patient Notice for Students in the Office

*See "When the Learner Arrives" on page 28.*

**To our patients:**

Our office is pleased to be participating in a supervised clinical learning program for medical students.

This type of education and training in places not associated with a medical school or hospital helps ensure that our future physicians will have the knowledge and experience they'll need for the "real world" of medical practice.

Your support of this program is helping train excellent doctors for the future.

Thank you.

## ❖ Patient Notice for Residents in the Office

*See "When the Learner Arrives" on page 28.*

**To our patients:**

Our office is pleased to be participating in a supervised clinical learning program for internal medicine residents (doctors who are training to be specialists in adult medicine).

This type of education and training in places not associated with a medical school or hospital helps ensure that our future physicians will have the knowledge and experience they'll need for the "real world" of medical practice.

Your support of this program is helping us train excellent doctors for the future.

Thank you.

## ❖ Biography of a Resident Physician
*To be made available in the office reception area.*
*See "When the Patients Arrive" on page 35.*

**New Resident Bio: Katie Smith, MD**

I grew up in Flint, Michigan, and graduated from Michigan State University where I studied art history and studio art. After receiving a fellowship in art history at the University of Michigan, I had the opportunity to live and study in Paris. After six months, however, I decided to return home to pursue a career in medicine, a decision that was strongly influenced by my father's illness.

I am a graduate of Michigan State University College of Human Medicine and now live in Grand Rapids, with my husband, Richard, and son, Bart. I am specializing in internal medicine and hope to practice here in Grand Rapids. My interests include traveling, cooking, skiing, and snorkeling.

## ❖ Educational Prescription Form
*See "Self-Directed (Indedpendent) Learning" on page 82.*

**Date and place to be filled** _____

**Patient's problem** _____

_____

_____

_____

_____

**Educational tasks to be completed before the session**

Learner: _____

Task: _____

**Presentation will cover:**
- ▶ How you found what you found
- ▶ What you found
- ▶ The validity and applicability of what you found
- ▶ How what you found will alter your management of the patient
- ▶ How well you think you did in filling this educational prescription

## ❖ Instructions To Help the Learner Organize the Patient Visit
*See "Strategies for Organizing the Office Visit" in on page 45.*

### Instructions for Students and Residents

Welcome to our office. We hope that you find providing care for patients in an office setting as enjoyable and as stimulating as we do. You will discover that outpatient care requires different skills from those you have learned practicing hospital medicine. The following paragraphs illustrate a few tips to help you begin.

A good patient visit requires effective organization of your time with the patient. Before all visits, mentally organize the encounter, including the time you spend with the patient. For return patients, remind yourself of the visit goal. You may want to review a visit plan with the preceptor before seeing the patient.

Begin the visit by setting mutual expectations about the agenda and the allotted time. Determine the patient's agenda for the visit with the question, "What concerns do you have today?" Limit the number of problems to two or three so they can be addressed within the allotted time. Prioritize problems by their severity, urgency, or importance to the patient, as appropriate. For return visits, state your agenda first, then ask for the patient's expectations. For example, you might say, "Mr. Smith, we have 20 minutes today. I'd like to follow up on your high blood pressure. Is there anything else you want to discuss?" If your and the patient's expectations do not match, negotiate how you are going to spend the time by saying something like, "That sounds like more than we will have time to discuss today. What two things are most important or pressing for you? We can address those issues today and set up another appointment to begin to address the others." This approach will satisfy most patients.

Patients appreciate when they know you are listening and including them in the planning. Determine what the patient thinks is going on and what they want done by asking, "What do *you* think is causing this? What do *you* think should be done?"

Early into the encounter, develop a favored initial hypothesis and consider its supporting evidence. Mentally create a weighted differential diagnosis and estimate the probability (low, medium, or high) of each. Consider the impact of not making an unlikely but important diagnosis emergently. For example, "In this patient, do I need to rule out ischemic heart disease as the cause of the chest pain even though it sounds like acid reflux?" Establish an initial focused action for each problem, including history, focused physical examination, tests, and treatment.

Office presentations are different from those performed in hospital wards. Many students and residents are taught to present as completely as possible, demonstrating their thoroughness. Other expectations include discussing all the patient's medical issues. Although these approaches are appropriate in some settings, the focus and time limitations in the office necessitate a different approach. The goals in the ambulatory setting are to emphasize the information needed for the patient's care *at this time* and to present as a concise summary to the preceptor as possible. The office presentation should begin with the patient identification, including whether her or she is a new or return patient and if the problem is acute or chronic. Next, give a statement of what questions *you* have as a result of your interaction with the patient. For example, "I am seeing a long-term patient of yours. He is 65 years old and was last seen three months ago for a cough that we attributed to a URI. He returns today because the cough persists. I have questions about where to go in his evaluation." Two other examples of prefacing your presentation with learning questions that need to be answered include: "I am seeing a 25-year-old woman, a new patient, who came in to establish care without any specific complaints. I had some questions about my findings on skin examination" and "Mr. Smith is a 40-year-old patient of yours who is here for pain medication for a migraine. I have questions about how to prescribe this medication for migraine headaches."

The patient identification and learner question is followed by a concise history of the presenting problems and a report of the focused physical examination. Do not report everything you know about the patient, only the pertinent positive and negative findings. (*Note:* You should know everything about the patient but you do not need tell the preceptor everything you know.) State your most likely diagnosis with brief supporting evidence. Include any diagnoses that you would not want to miss (e.g., worst-case scenarios) and their likelihood. Present your plan with brief supporting evidence. State it as best you can, recognizing that parts may hinge on the question(s) you need answered. Discuss your question and plan with the preceptor. Prepare the follow-up.

Patient education should be concise and clear enough that the patient can go home and explain to a friend or family member "what the doctor said." Assess the patient's level of understanding by asking questions, for example, "I think your skin rash is most likely due to psoriasis. Have you heard of psoriasis? What do you know about psoriasis?" Based on the patient's response, direct your education accordingly. Avoid the use of medical jargon (e.g., use "rash" instead of "lesions").

If the patient brings up a problem at the end of the visit ("I forgot to mention my back pain"), do not despair. Quickly assess and triage the situation to an immediate evaluation versus following up with it at the next visit. In assessing the seriousness of the condition, it may be helpful to consider why the patient did not mention it earlier. Was it because he or she is afraid of its seriousness, is simply being complete, or is truly just remembering it? Also, the patient may not want closure and is not ready for you to leave. Ask the preceptor for help if you are unsure if a problem needs to be evaluated emergently.

## ❖ Tools To Help the Learner Organize the Patient Visit
### *What?—The Patient's Agenda*
"What should we talk about today?"
### *Why?—The Patient's Attribution*

| Problem 1 | Problem 2 | Problem 3 |
|---|---|---|
|  |  |  |

"What do you think is causing this? What do you think should be done?"
### *Why?—The Favored Initial Hypothesis*

| Problem 1 | Problem 2 | Problem 3 |
|---|---|---|
|  |  |  |

| Problem 1 | Problem 2 | Problem 3 |
|---|---|---|
|  |  |  |
| Supporting Evidence | Supporting Evidence | Supporting Evidence |
|  |  |  |

### *What Else?—The Differential Diagnosis*
Estimate probability "[P]" as being "L" (low), "M" (medium), or "H" (high)
### *What Now?—Initial Focused Actions*

| Problem 1 | Problem 2 | Problem 3 |
|---|---|---|
| [P]= | [P]= | [P]= |
| [P]= | [P]= | [P]= |
| [P]= | [P]= | [P]= |

| Problem 1 | Problem 2 | Problem 3 |
|---|---|---|
| History: | History: | History: |
| Exam: | Exam: | Exam: |
| Tests: | Tests: | Tests: |
| Therapy: | Therapy: | Therapy: |

## ❖ Patient Presentation Format for Learners

*See "Strategies for Organizing the Office Visit" on page 45.*

### Identifying Data and Chief Complaint

❑ Patient name

❑ Age

❑ New or return visit (last seen _____ )

❑ Questions from the last visit that need to be addressed

❑ New questions for today

### Questions Needing Answers (General)

❑ Diagnostic uncertainty

❑ History to ask

❑ Pertinent examination to perform

❑ Verify examination findings

❑ Further evaluation

❑ Treatment

❑ Follow-up

❑ Social services

### Concise History of Present Illness

❑ Include only pertinent positive and negative findings

❑ History

❑ Past medical history

❑ Social history

❑ Family history

### Concise Physical Examination

❑ Only pertinent positive and negative findings

❑ Most likely diagnosis

❑ Provide brief supporting evidence

❑ Estimate likelihood

❑ Include any "wouldn't-want-to-miss" diagnoses

❑ Your plan may depend on answers to your questions

## *Questions Needing Answers (Specific)*

❑ Diagnostic questions
❑ Treatment plan
❑ Plans for follow-up

## ❖ Generic Acute Patient Script
(See "Data Collection and Patient Presentation" on page 45)

| | |
|---|---|
| **Acute Focused History** | acute problem |

1. **Character/circumstance**
   Including patient concerns

2. **Location**

3. **Exacerbating/alleviating factors**
   Alternative medicine, prescription or
   OTC meds, position, activity, etc.

4. **Radiation**

5. **Associated symptoms**
   Must have a differential diagnosis in
   mind so you can ask about symptoms
   relevant to that differential

6. **Severity**
   Limit of function, interference with
   sleep; scale from 1-10

7. **Timing/pattern**
   Acute vs. chronic, constant vs. intermit-
   tent, accelerating. **Each** symptom needs
   a timeline. Why presenting today?

   *Onset:*
   Sudden, gradual. **Duration** of each
   episode and total duration of problem

   *Relevant past medical histo
   ry:*
   Including **allergies** and current medications

   *Relevant social history:*
   Tobacco use, alcohol, occupation, travel,
   hobbies may be relevant. Does patient
   live alone?

   *Relevant family history:*
   Familial disorders that may relate to the

## ❖ Generic Chronic Patient Script
(See "Data Collection and Patient Presentation" on page 45)

### Focused Chronic Illness History

1. **Interval history**
2. **Compliance**
   - Diet
   - Medications
   - Exercise if relevant
   - Special (i.e., elevating legs or wearing support stocking for edema)
3. **Symptoms** that might be associated with the problem.

   Much of your job in medical school is to learn what symptoms go with what problems.

   Pattern recognition is crucial in clinical care.

   **Anticipated possible complications**
   Complications of the illness itself and anticipated possible complications from treatment, including medications:
   - Side effects
   - Adverse drug reactions
   - Drug-disease
   - Drug-drug interactions

   Use a drug reference to check for side effects for any drug the patient is on.
4. Can you and the patient think of how to **avoid complications in future**?

### Focused Chronic Illness Physical Exam

1. **Vital signs** always
2. **General appearance**
3. **Remainder of exam** is focused on the problems (i.e., for hypertension consider whether you need to check for anticipated complications like heart failure).

   *Think about checking:*

   - Fundi
   - Cardiovascular: inspection for ectopic impulses, palpation for carotid, PMI, ectopic impulses, auscultation: S1 and S2, S3 or S4 gallops, murmurs
   - Abdomen: ascites, hepatojugular reflux if thinking about failure
   - Extremities: edema, peripheral pulses (if concerned about complication of peripheral vascular disease)
   - Remember, the physical examination is often therapeutic as well as diagnostic.

## ❖ Feedback Note Organized According to Competencies
(See "Time-Saving Tips for Giving Feedback" on page 104 in Chapter 8)

| | |
|---|---|
| **Student Name** | |
| **Rotation Dates** | |
| **Patient Care-Gathering Historical Information** (includes gathering all aspects of history and other patient data) | ☐ Well done<br>☐ Needs Improvement<br>Specify Skill Observed:<br>Feedback Note: |
| **Patient Care-Physical Examination Skills** (includes correctly performing appropriate exams) | ☐ Well done<br>☐ Needs Improvement<br>Specify Skill Observed:<br>Feedback Note: |
| **Patient Care-Diagnostic Skills** (includes ability to generate and support a prioritized differential diagnosis) | ☐ Well done<br>☐ Needs Improvement<br>Specify Skill Observed:<br>Feedback Note: |
| **Patient Care-Management Skills** (includes planing next diagnostic tests or therapeutic intervention) | ☐ Well done<br>☐ Needs Improvement<br>Specify Skill Observed:<br>Feedback Note: |
| **Medical Knowledge** (includes epidemiological, behavioral, and clinical) | ☐ Well done<br>☐ Needs Improvement<br>Feedback Note: |
| **Interpersonal and Communication Skills: Patients** (includes interviews, counseling, education) | ☐ Well done<br>☐ Needs Improvement<br>Specify Skill Observed:<br>Feedback Note: |
| **Interpersonal and Communication Skills: Professional Associates** (includes case reports, working relationships, team work) | ☐ Well done<br>☐ Needs Improvement<br>Specify Skill Observed:<br>Feedback Note: |
| **Professionalism** (includes ethical behavior, responsibility, respect, compassion, integrity) | ☐ Well done<br>☐ Needs Improvement<br>Specify Behavior Observed:<br>Feedback Note: |
| **Practice-Based Improvement** (retrieval and appraisal of scientific evidence, performance measures, quality improvement) | ☐ Well done<br>☐ Needs Improvement<br>Specify Behavior Observed:<br>Feedback Note: |
| **Systems-Based Practice** (effective use and coordination of includes ancillary services, office management) | ☐ Well done<br>☐ Needs Improvement<br>Specify Behavior Observed:<br>Feedback Note: |

## ❖ Mini-CEX Form
(See "Basic Steps in the Evaluation Process" on page 106 in Chapter 8)

### Guidelines For Implementing the Mini-CEX

The mini-clinical evaluation exercise (CEX) focuses on the core skills that residents demonstrate in patient encounters. It can be easily implemented by attending physicians as a routine, seamless evaluation of residents in any setting. The mini-CEX is a 15-20 minute observation or "snapshot" of a resident/patient interaction. Based on multiple encounters over time, this method provides a valid, reliable measure of residents' performance. *Attending physicians are encouraged to perform one mini-CEX per resident during the rotation.*

**Settings to Conduct Mini-CEX**
In-patient services
  (CCU/ICU, Ward)
Ambulatory
Emergency Department
Other including admission, discharge

**Mini-CEX Evaluators**
Attending Physicians
Supervising Physicians
Chief Residents
Senior Residents

**Forms and Rating Scale:** Packet includes 10 forms; after completing form, provide "original" to program director and "copy" to resident. Nine point rating scale is used; rating of 4 is defined as *"marginal"* and conveys the expectation that with remediation the resident will meet the standards for Board certification.

Descriptors of Competencies Demonstrated During the Mini-CEX

**Medical Interviewing Skills:** Facilitates patient's telling of story; effectively uses questions/directions to obtain accurate, adequate information needed; responds appropriately to affect, non-verbal cues.

**Physical Examination Skills:** Follows efficient, logical sequence; balances screening/diagnostic steps for problem; informs patient; sensitive to patient's comfort, modesty.

**Humanistic Qualities/Professionalism:** Shows respect, compassion, empathy, establishes trust; attends to patient's needs of comfort, modesty, confidentiality, information.

**Clinical Judgment:** Selectively orders/performs appropriate diagnostic studies, considers risks, benefits.

**Counseling Skills:** Explains rationale for test/treatment, obtains patient's consent, educates/counsels regarding management.

**Organization/Efficiency:** Prioritizes, is timely; succinct.

**Overall Clinical Competence:** Demonstrates judgment, synthesis, caring, effectiveness, efficiency.

*If you have any questions, please call ABIM at 1-800-441-2246*

# Mini-Clinical Evaluation Exercise (CEX)

**Evaluator:** _____    **Date:** _____

**Resident:** _____    ☐ R-1   ☐ R-2   ☐ R-3

**Patient Problem/Dx:** _____

| | | | |
|---|---|---|---|
| **Setting:** | ☐ Ambulatory | ☐ In-Patient   ☐ ED | ☐ Other _____ |
| **Patient:** | Age: _____ | Sex: _____   ☐ New | ☐ Follow-up |
| **Complexity:** | | ☐ Low   ☐ Moderate | ☐ High |
| **Focus:** | ☐ Data Gathering | ☐ Diagnosis   ☐ Therapy | ☐ Counseling |

**1. Medical Interviewing Skills**    (☐ Not Observed)

| 1 | 2 | 3 | 4 | 5 | 6 | 7 | 8 | 9 |
|---|---|---|---|---|---|---|---|---|
| | UNSATIFACTORY | | | SATISFACTORY | | | SUPERIOR | |

**2. Physical Examination Skills**    (☐ Not Observed)

| 1 | 2 | 3 | 4 | 5 | 6 | 7 | 8 | 9 |
|---|---|---|---|---|---|---|---|---|
| | UNSATIFACTORY | | | SATISFACTORY | | | SUPERIOR | |

**3. Humanistic Qualities/Professionalism**

| 1 | 2 | 3 | 4 | 5 | 6 | 7 | 8 | 9 |
|---|---|---|---|---|---|---|---|---|
| | UNSATIFACTORY | | | SATISFACTORY | | | SUPERIOR | |

**4. Clinical Judgment**    (☐ Not Observed)

| 1 | 2 | 3 | 4 | 5 | 6 | 7 | 8 | 9 |
|---|---|---|---|---|---|---|---|---|
| | UNSATIFACTORY | | | SATISFACTORY | | | SUPERIOR | |

**5. Counseling Skills**    (☐ Not Observed)

| 1 | 2 | 3 | 4 | 5 | 6 | 7 | 8 | 9 |
|---|---|---|---|---|---|---|---|---|
| | UNSATIFACTORY | | | SATISFACTORY | | | SUPERIOR | |

**6. Organization/Efficiency**    (☐ Not Observed)

| 1 | 2 | 3 | 4 | 5 | 6 | 7 | 8 | 9 |
|---|---|---|---|---|---|---|---|---|
| | UNSATIFACTORY | | | SATISFACTORY | | | SUPERIOR | |

**7. Overall Clinical Competency**    (☐ Not Observed)

| 1 | 2 | 3 | 4 | 5 | 6 | 7 | 8 | 9 |
|---|---|---|---|---|---|---|---|---|
| | UNSATIFACTORY | | | SATISFACTORY | | | SUPERIOR | |

**Mini-CEX Time:   Observing _____ Minutes   Providing Feedback: _____ Minutes**

Evaluator Satisfaction with Mini-CEX
LOW   1   2   3   4   5   6   7   8   9   HIGH

Resident Satisfaction with Mini-CEX
LOW   1   2   3   4   5   6   7   8   9   HIGH

Comments: _____

_____

_____

_____    _____
Resident Signature                            Evaluator Signature

## ❖ Patient Satisfaction Form
*See Chapter 8, Learner Feedback and Evaluation, on page 97.*

| This Doctor: | Strongly Disagree → | | | Strongly Agree |
|---|---|---|---|---|
| Follows through on problems | 1 | 2 | 3 | 4 | 5 |
| Is truthful and honest with me without avoiding the issues | 1 | 2 | 3 | 4 | 5 |
| Is in a hurry | 1 | 2 | 3 | 4 | 5 |
| Expresses concern for my feelings and needs, not just my physical status | 1 | 2 | 3 | 4 | 5 |
| Comforts or reassures me and my family | 1 | 2 | 3 | 4 | 5 |
| Asks me how I am doing | 1 | 2 | 3 | 4 | 5 |
| Keeps his or her promises to me | 1 | 2 | 3 | 4 | 5 |
| Pays attention to concerns and requests that I feel are important | 1 | 2 | 3 | 4 | 5 |
| Explains and clarifies information for me | 1 | 2 | 3 | 4 | 5 |
| Answers my questions | 1 | 2 | 3 | 4 | 5 |
| Makes uncaring remarks or does things I find offensive | 1 | 2 | 3 | 4 | 5 |
| Discusses the options for my treatment | 1 | 2 | 3 | 4 | 5 |
| Uses terms that I can understand | 1 | 2 | 3 | 4 | 5 |
| Includes me in decisions and choices about my care | 1 | 2 | 3 | 4 | 5 |
| Arranges for adequate privacy when examining or talking with me | 1 | 2 | 3 | 4 | 5 |
| Has a neat, clean, well-groomed appearance | 1 | 2 | 3 | 4 | 5 |
| Is short-tempered or abrupt with my family or me | 1 | 2 | 3 | 4 | 5 |
| Does not rush or spend too little time with me | 1 | 2 | 3 | 4 | 5 |
| Asks if I need anything or what he or she can do for me | 1 | 2 | 3 | 4 | 5 |
| Asks how I want to be addressed, then greets me in that way | 1 | 2 | 3 | 4 | 5 |
| Seems knowledgeable and concerned about my case and me | 1 | 2 | 3 | 4 | 5 |
| Asks questions about my symptoms | 1 | 2 | 3 | 4 | 5 |
| Treats me in too intimate or personal a manner | 1 | 2 | 3 | 4 | 5 |
| Asks me how I feel about my problems | 1 | 2 | 3 | 4 | 5 |

Republished with permission from Weaver MJ, Ow CL, Walker DJ, Degenhardt EF. A questionnaire for patients' evaluations of their physicians humanistic behaviors. *J Gen Intern Med.* 1993;8:135–9.

## ❖ Behaviorally Anchored RIME Evaluation Form
(See "What Is An Educator?" on page 114 in Chapter 8)

| Skill Area | Area for Improvement | Competent | Strength |
|---|---|---|---|
| **Reporting** | Data gathering and reporting are incomplete or disorganized. Rarely incorporates test results or other data (e.g., nursing information). Incomplete or incompetent physical exam. | Gathers pertinent data, reports in an organized fashion. Utilizes lab results, etc. Competent physical exam skills; occasionally will miss findings. | Data complete and concise, presentations and write-ups are organized. Always uses test results and other pertinent data. Physical examination thorough, focussed when appropriate, and reliable. |
| **Interpretation** | Rarely/occasionally able to generate a differential including most likely and do not miss. Difficulty justifying/demonstrating clinical reasoning. | Usually generates a good differential including most likely and do not miss diagnoses. Justifies/demonstrates clinical reasoning when prompted. | Consistently generates a good differential including most likely and do not miss. Justifies/demonstrates clinical reasoning without prompting. |
| **Management** | Rarely able to suggest appropriate tests or therapy. Relies on preceptor almost exclusively. | Almost always able to suggest appropriate tests or therapy. Looks up questions. | Consistently orders appropriate tests and therapy. Incorporates outside reading. |
| **Education** | Rarely does outside reading or incorporates it into patient care. Knowledge base concerns. Relies on preceptor for learning. Rarely self-directed. | Almost always reads basic texts and specialty texts when needed. Teaches preceptors something occasionally. Mostly self-directed. Can apply evidence-based medicine concepts. | Practices evidence-based medicine independently using primary and secondary sources. Summarizes information for colleagues. Teaches preceptor something frequently. |
| **Interpersonal skills** | Often poor rapport with patients and colleagues, disorganized, disrespectful. Rarely able to demonstrate empathy. | Respectful, good rapport with patients and colleagues. Able to demonstrate empathy. | Always respectful. Excellent rapport with patients and colleagues. Regularly demonstrates empathy. |
| **Professionalism** | Sometimes unprofessional, leaves work undone. Sometimes unprepared. Does the minimum. | Prompt, appropriate. Follows through on patient care and educational issues. | Always prompt, well prepared, and professional. Does patient care follow-up without prompting. Is self-directed. |

## ❖ Questions Used to Teach and Evaluate Learners

| Type | Examples | Comments |
|---|---|---|
| **Factual** | Who is the patient? Why is the patient here? When did the patient's back pain begin? What is the most common cause of back pain? | Factual questions, for obtaining information and beginning discussions, consist of the five "W"s: who, what, when, where and why. If you find yourself using only factual questions, it probably means you haven't done an adequate job of orienting the student to your presentation needs or the learner hasn't mastered the technique; either way, go back to square one and reassess the process. |
| **Broadening** | What are some other causes of back pain? | Broadening questions can be used to assess additional knowledge not elicited by factual questions. This is a useful type of question, but having to use it suggests either that the student wasn't asked to provide a differential diagnosis as part of the presentation or that he or she has not mastered this skill. *Refer the student to the "Patient Presentation Format for Learners" on page 126.* Consider whether you still want the student to present a differential diagnosis for each patient; follow up with the appropriate instructions. |
| **Justifying** | What in the patient's history and physical examination supports your diagnosis? | Justifying questions are used to challenge ideas and assess depth of knowledge and understanding. These are excellent probing questions suggested by the microskills teaching model. |
| **Hypothetical** | Suppose your patient has a history of prostate cancer. How would that influence your diagnosis? | Hypothetical questions are used to explore new situations and are effective in creating a more diverse patient population for the learner. This type of question can be useful when seeing your tenth patient with a "run of the mill" problem by allowing you to create new learning situations. |
| **Alternative** | Suppose we got an MRI scan next week instead of today. What would be the advantages and disadvantages? | Alternative questions can be used to assess decision-making skills by presenting different plans and asking for probable outcomes. Answering this type of question requires a higher order of content mastery and judgment. |

# APPENDIX B

## Summaries and Checklists
## for Preceptors

## ❖ Before the Learner Arrives Preparatory Checklist

*See "Before the Learner Arrives" on page 25.*

### *One Week Before the Learner Arrives*

❑ Review the institution's learning goals and objectives

❑ Review the institution's orientation materials

❑ Review the student's information or application (if available)

❑ Have a reliable number for the institution's contact person in case of problems

❑ Have staff confirm the dates and times of the instruction in your office with the sponsoring institution

❑ Send any information the learner should know about the practice to the sponsoring institution for distribution to the learner

❑ Schedule a 30-minute orientation for the learner

❑ Schedule time at the end of the experience for learner evaluation and feedback

❑ Consider making a brochure or handout for patients about the learner (*see "Biography of a Resident Physician" on page 130*)

❑ Consider altering your schedule for the precepting experience (*see "Patient Scheduling" on page 31*)

### *Two to Three Days Before the Learner Arrives*

❑ Remind staff and partners of the impending arrival of the learner

❑ Distribute copy of the learner's application or personal information (if available) to staff and partners

❑ Brief the staff on the learner's responsibilities

❑ Review with the staff their role with the learner

❑ Coach the staff on how to present the learner to patients

❑ Identify a parking place for the learner

❑ Identify a workspace for the learner

❑ Equip workspace with needed references, paper, and writing utensils

❑ Gather forms (e.g., laboratory, physical therapy, radiology, consultation) for learner orientation

❑ Generate list of staff, their office locations, and a short description of their responsibilities (save in file)

❑ Make copies of patient notices about the learner for reception area (*see "Patient Notice for Students in the Office" and "Patient Notice for Residents in the Office" on pages 128 and 129*)

❑ Make a list of what to cover during learner orientation (save in file; *see "When the Learner Arrives Orientation Checklist" on page 150*)

❑ If the learner will dictate notes, prepare instructions (save in file)

## ❖ When the Learner Arrives Orientation Checklist
*See "When the Learner Arrives" on page 28.*

❑ Post notices in the reception area about the learner

❑ Have the receptionist inform patients about the learner

❑ Review with the learner the institution's learning goals and objectives

❑ Review the "Clinical Skills Inventory" with learner (*see "Previous Experiences" on page 28*)

❑ Review the learner's expectations for this experience

❑ Review your expectations for the experience

❑ Consider signing a learning contract with learner (*see "Learner Contract" on page 126*)

❑ Review working hours

❑ Review days off

❑ Review potential schedule conflicts and attempt to resolve them

❑ Review how to contact office in case of personal emergency or unanticipated schedule conflict

❑ Review office rules and policies (e.g., parking, dress code, meals, telephone and computer use)

❑ Orient the learner to his or her personal workspace

❑ Review contents of examination room and where equipment, supplies, and forms are located

❑ Introduce learner to staff (including their responsibilities) and to partners

❑ Review when and how teaching will occur

❑ Review when and how feedback will be provided

❑ Review scheduling and which patients the learner will see

❑ Review how much time should be spent with patients

❑ Review what parts of examination should and should not be done in your absence

❑ Review how to organize the learner's time with the patient and you (*see "Strategies for Organizing the Office Visit" on page 45*)

❑ Review how you want patients presented to you (*see "Patient Presentation Format for Learners" on page 137*)

❑ Review how you want notes written or dictated

❑ Review which clinical tests are performed in the office

❑ Review how to order imaging studies and other diagnostic tests

❑ Review how to schedule a consultation

❑ Review how to schedule a follow-up appointment

❑ Review where to retrieve patient education materials

❑ Review how to retrieve test results

❑ Review how to request a patient chart

❑ Review when the final evaluation will take place

❑ Review how to handle an office emergency (e.g., cardiac arrest)

## ❖ The Wave Schedule

*See "Patient Scheduling" on page 31.*

WAVE SCHEDULE

| Time (AM) | Original Physician Schedule | Learner Wave Schedule | Physician Wave Schedule |
|---|---|---|---|
| | | Patient A | |
| 8:00–8:20 | Patient A | Patient A | Patient B |
| 8:20–8:40 | Patient B | Writes note | Patient A |
| 840–9:00 | Patient C | Patient D | Patient C |
| 9:00–9:20 | Patient D | Patient D | Patient E |
| 9:20–9:40 | Patient E | Writes note | Patient D |
| 9:40–10:00 | Patient F | Patient G | Patient F |
| 10:00–10:20 | Patient G | Patient G | Patient H |
| 10:20–10:40 | Patient H | Writes note | Patient G |
| 10:40–11:00 | Patient I | Patient J | Patient I |
| 11:00–11:20 | Patient J | Patient J | Patient K |
| 11:20–11:40 | Patient K | Writes note | Patient J |
| 11:40–Noon | Patient L | | Patient L |

- ▶ This model allows physicians to see the same number of patients promptly with a learner present
- ▶ The wave schedule can be more intense for advanced learners
- ▶ The wave schedule can be less intense for the novice learner
- ▶ This model is easily adaptable to schedules of any appointment length, provided that the slots are of equal length

## ❖ When the Patients Arrive Checklist

*See "When the Patients Arrive" on page 35.*

❑ Have the receptionist inform patients that you have a learner in the office today

❑ Distribute brochure or handout about the learner to patients, if available (*see "Biography of a Resident Physician" on page 130*)

❑ Ask the patient's permission before bringing a learner into the examination room

   ► Couch your request positively, e.g., "I have a medical student/resident working with me today. If it's okay with you, I'd like him/her to talk to you and examine you first. I will come in and see you afterwards."

❑ If you teach frequently, inform new patients that you work with learners

❑ Have the office staff inform you about any positive or negative feedback from the patients about the learner

❑ Consider measuring your patients' satisfaction with the learner by using the *"Patient Satisfaction Form" on page 144*

## ❖ Summary of the Learning Experience

❑ Expose the learner to all the things you do as a physician and as a member of the community
- ▶ How you relate to other specialists and medical professionals
- ▶ How you keep up on medical knowledge
- ▶ What you do in the hospital and in other settings
- ▶ Your participation in professional organizations
- ▶ Your civic and community activities

❑ Require novice learners to observe you with selected patients performing various skills
- ▶ Taking a focused history
- ▶ Performing part of an examination
- ▶ Performing a procedure
- ▶ Counseling a patient

❑ Provide opportunities for the learner to see patients first (alone)
- ▶ Take the history
- ▶ Perform the examination
- ▶ Form their own impressions about diagnosis
- ▶ Generate a management plan
- ▶ Report to you
- ▶ Write the orders
- ▶ Write the prescription
- ▶ Arrange for follow-up

❑ Organize the visit for the learner (*see "Tools To Help the Learner Organize the Patient Visit" on page 135*)
- ▶ "Prime" the learner by providing pertinent patient-specific background information, e.g., "Mrs. Jones is a healthy 28-year-old woman and is here for her yearly examination. At her age, what are the important screening issues to be covered?"
- ▶ "Frame" the visit by focusing on what should be accomplished at this visit and how long it should take, e.g., "This patient has several problems, but today I'd like you to focus on the patient's care of her diabetes. Spend 15 minutes taking the history and then come find me."

❑ Familiarize yourself with the common models of case-based learning (*see Chapter 5*)
  ▶ Microskills model
  ▶ "Aunt Minnie" model
  ▶ Modeling Problem Solving
  ▶ The One-Minute Observation
  ▶ Learner-Centered Precepting
  ▶ SNAPPS Precepting Model
❑ Set "mini-goals"
❑ Consider strategies to improve teaching efficiency (*see Chapter 6*)
  ▶ Consider a wave schedule (*see "Patient Scheduling" on page 31 and "The Wave Schedule" on pages 32 and 152*)
  ▶ Have the learner present the case in front of the patient in the examination room
  ▶ Encourage collaborative examinations
  ▶ Use the technique of active observation (*see "Active Observation" on page 79 and "Summary of Active Observation" on page 161*), e.g., "Let's counsel this patient about quitting smoking. Watch my approach. I'd like you to review this [brief chapter or paper] and try to counsel the next patient with this problem."
  ▶ Expose the learner to educational experiences beyond patient care
  ▶ Expose the learner to service-based education
  ▶ Have the learner keep notes of questions to be discussed at the end of the day
  ▶ Have the learner engage in "Self-Directed (Independent) Learning" (*see page 82 and "Summary of Self-Directed [Independent] Learning" on page 162*)
❑ Ending the day
  ▶ Meet with the learner to discuss unanswered questions or concerns
  ▶ Encourage independent learning by assigning "homework"
  ▶ Follow up with learner on any "homework" assignments
  ▶ Consider using the "Educational Prescription Form" (*see page 131*)
❑ Feedback and evaluation (*see Chapter 8*)
  ▶ Provide frequent, timely feedback
  ▶ Base evaluation on evidence
  ▶ Consider using the "RIME Evaluation Framework" (*see page 112 and "Summary of RIME Evaluation Framework" on page 166*)

## ❖ Summary of the Microskills Model for Precepting

*See "The Microskills Model" on page 52.*

❑ Get a commitment
  ▶ Ask the learner to commit to some decision or plan of action, e.g., "What do you think is going on with this patient?"
❑ Probe for supporting evidence
  ▶ Ask the learner for the evidence that supports the commitment, e.g., "What were the major findings that led you to that diagnosis?", "Why did you choose medication X rather than medication Y?"
❑ Teach general rules
  ▶ Teaching is more memorable and more easily transferable to other cases when it is offered as a general rule rather than as a patient-specific plan, e.g., "In a young patient with mechanical low back pain, an X-ray is not needed initially."
❑ Reinforce what was done right
  ▶ Provide positive, explicit, behavior-specific feedback, e.g., "You were very empathic with that patient, and she responded by providing important information in the history."
  ▶ Positive feedback is not general praise, e.g., "You did a good job with that last patient."
❑ Correct mistakes
  ▶ Attempt to frame the mistake as being "not the best" rather than "bad" or "wrong."
  ▶ Provide specific guidance on improvement, e.g., "You might be more successful next time this happens if you try..."

## ❖ Summary of the "Aunt Minnie" Model of Precepting

*See "The 'Aunt Minnie' Model" on page 60.*

❑ Have the learner collect data from the patient
  ▶ If the patient problem is straightforward, the learner informs the preceptor that he or she has an "Aunt Minnie" case
  ▶ If the patient problem is not straightforward, then either the preceptor uses the microskills or other case-based teaching model
❑ The learner presents only the chief complaint and probable diagnosis (30 seconds)
❑ Learner and preceptor focus on patient management issues
❑ Have the learner write the note
❑ Examine the patient without the learner present
❑ Provide feedback to the learner by doing one of the following:
  ▶ Confirm the diagnosis
  ▶ Provide the correct diagnosis (1–5 minutes)
❑ Review the learner's written note

## ❖ Summary of the One-Minute Observation
*See "The One-Minute Observation" on page 63.*

❑ Explain the purpose of the observation to the learner
❑ Explain how the observation will occur
❑ Select one skill for observation
❑ Inform the patient of what will take place
❑ Observe for a brief period of time without interrupting
❑ Leave the room and have the learner join you when finished with the patient
❑ Provide immediate feedback on what you observed
❑ Use the information gained to plan your teaching
❑ Repeat the process observing other skills
❑ Evaluate the learner's skills over time, using multiple, brief periods of observation

## ❖ Summary of Learner-Centered Precepting

*See "Learner-Centered Precepting" on page 64.*

### *Identification*

❑ Learner presents patient
- ▶ Gives name and age
- ▶ Specifies whether the patient is new or a return
- ▶ Details chief complaint
- ▶ Identifies teaching need, e.g., "My question is, should Mrs. Smith have an insulin pump?"

### *Information*

❑ Learner presents patient data, diagnosis, and plan
- ▶ Gives concise history
- ▶ Details pertinent examination findings
- ▶ Determines most likely diagnosis
- ▶ Develops treatment plan

### *Issues*

❑ Learner formulates specific questions needed to care for patient
- ▶ Verification of findings
- ▶ Content (knowledge) information
- ▶ Logistical information

## ❖ Summary of the SNAPPS Precepting Model

*(See "SNAPPS Model of Learner-Centered Precepting" on page 66)*

- ❑ **S**ummarize briefly the history and findings
- ❑ **N**arrow the differential to two or three possibilities
- ❑ **A**nalyze the differential by comparing and contrasting the possibilities
- ❑ **P**robe the preceptor by asking questions about uncertainties, difficulties, or alternative approaches
- ❑ **P**lan management for the patient's medical issues
- ❑ **S**elect a case-related issue for self-directed learning

## ❖ Summary of Active Observation

*See "Active Observation" on page 79.*

❏ Explain the rationale for the observation, e.g., "You should watch me do this because you need help with cardiac auscultation"

❏ Tell the learner what to observe, e.g., "Notice how I listen to the patient's heart in several positions and use both the bell and diaphragm."

❏ Ask the learner should review with you what was observed, e.g., "Tell me how I examined the heart"

❏ Tell the learner to practice the skill just demonstrated, e.g., "When you see the next patient, I want you to practice cardiac auscultation"

❏ Give feedback to the learner on how he or she performed the skill

❏ *Important Point:* Active observation is not simply "shadowing"; it should be performed with well-defined learner goals and accountabilities

## ❖ Summary of Self-Directed (Independent) Learning

*See "Self-Directed (Independent) Learning" on page 82.*

### Identify the Need

❑ After hearing the patient presentation (or at the end of the session), have the learner either identify his or her learning question or prompt him or her by asking
  ▶ "Based on the patients you saw today, what are your questions?"
  ▶ "What is the one thing you would like to learn more about?"
  ▶ "What troubled you today?"
  ▶ "What might you improve?"

### Make an Assignment

❑ Ask the learner to formulate the question
❑ Ask the learner to research the answer to the question
❑ Specify a time for the learner to report back to you with the results of the research

### Identify Potential Resources

❑ Textbooks (print and electronic)
❑ MEDLINE or other databases
❑ Journal articles
❑ Consultants

### "Close the Loop"

❑ The learner reports back on what was found
  ▶ Gives an oral presentation
  ▶ Submits a written outline
  ▶ Incorporates it into a patient write-up or assessment
❑ Consider using the "Educational Prescription Form" (*see page 129*) to facilitate the learning

## ❖ Teaching Procedural Skills

*See "Teaching Procedures in the Office", Chapter 7.*

1. Define the skill to be taught
2. Create learning objectives
3. Write a description of the skill
   - List steps and sub-steps
   - Organize steps in proper sequence
   - Create a checklist for the skill
4. Motivate the learner
5. Review past experiences with the skill
6. Provide a concise overview
7. Demonstrate the skill
   - Name each essential step as it is performed
   - Focus on correct performance and quality indicators
8. Commit steps to memory (consider using code names for each step)
9. Practice (simulation first, if possible)
   - Observe and prompt learner
   - Provide feedback
10. Perfecting
    - Provide increasingly difficult or different practice situations
    - Elaborate finer points
11. Document proficiency

## ❖ Summary of Feedback Tips

*See "Feedback Tips" on page 99 in Chapter 8.*

❑ Set expectation for feedback
❑ Provide ongoing and frequent feedback
❑ Provide timely and specific feedback
❑ Explain the consequences of the observed behavior
❑ Limit amount of feedback in any one session
❑ Focus feedback on behavior, not personality
❑ Focus feedback on behavior that can change
❑ Offer tips for future behavior

## ❖ Summary of Evaluation

*See Chapter 8, Learner Feedback and Evaluation, on page 97.*

❑ Summative evaluation occurs at the end of instruction
  ▶ Review the learner's past performance
  ▶ Base your review on the sponsoring institution's evaluation criteria
❑ The final evaluation should never be a surprise to the learner
  ▶ Avoid surprise by providing specific feedback periodically throughout the precepting experience
❑ Consider referring to the "RIME Evaluation Framework" (*see page 112 and "Summary of RIME Evaluation Framework" on page 166*) before evaluating the learner
  ▶ Base the evaluation on systematic, first-hand observations of the learner's performance
❑ Emphasize changes in behavior and performance that will lead to the desired competencies
❑ Deliver the evaluation in oral and written forms
❑ Make a copy of your evaluation and file it
❑ Return the written evaluation to the sponsoring institution on time
❑ Avoid rating errors when filling out the written evaluation form
  ▶ *The "halo/horn" effect:* Basing your evaluation on reports of previous performance
  ▶ *Restriction of range:* Using the same rating for all components of the evaluation, rather than rating each individually
  ▶ *Rating nonperformance attributes:* Taking into consideration behavior attributes when rating nonbehavioral qualities
❑ Schedule time for the evaluation when you will not be interrupted or hurried
❑ Begin the evaluation by having the learner perform a self-assessment
❑ Consider having the learner fill out a copy of the final evaluation form provided by the institution before your meeting
❑ Use the learner's self-evaluation to begin the discussion of your own observations

## ❖ Summary of the RIME Evaluation Framework

*See "The RIME Evaluation Framework" on page 112.*

### Reporter

❑ One who can efficiently and accurately collect patient data

❑ One who can recognize normal from abnormal

❑ One who can identify and label new problems

❑ One who can communicate collected data orally and in writing

### Interpreter

❑ One who can prioritize problems

❑ One who can follow up and interpret abnormal findings and tests

❑ One who can create a differential diagnosis

❑ One who can prioritize a differential diagnosis

### Manager

❑ One who can determine when action is necessary

❑ One who can choose the most appropriate diagnostic test

❑ One who can choose the most appropriate management strategy

❑ One who can customize a plan according to patient circumstances and preferences

### Educator

❑ One who can identify knowledge gaps and develop plans to address them

❑ One who can share new knowledge with others

❑ One who can understand the use and limits of evidence in the care of patients

# ❖ Summary of the GRADE Strategy for Evaluation*

*See "Evaluation Using the GRADE Strategy" on page 111 in Chapter 8.*

| |
|---|
| **G – Get Ready** (see Before the Learner Arrives, on page 25)<br>• Review course expectations and the evaluation form<br>• Articulate your expectations for the learner<br>• Schedule the end-of-experience evaluation meeting |
| **R – Review expectations with the learner** (see Before the Learner Arrives, on page 25)<br>• Meet with the learner early in the experience<br>• Determine the learner's knowledge and skill level (see Summary of the Learning Experience, on page 154)<br>• Review the programs goals, your goals, and the learner's goals<br>• Describe the evaluation process |
| **A – Assess** (see Learner Feedback and Evaluation, Chapter 8)<br>• Observe<br>• Record<br>• Provide feedback regularly<br>• Have learner self-assess |
| **D – Discuss assessment** (see Learner Feedback and Evaluation, Chapter 8)<br>• Formal meeting<br>• Learner and preceptor fill out evaluation forms<br>• Compare evaluations together<br>• Discuss differences and whether expectations were met |
| **E – End with a grade** (see Learner Feedback and Evaluation, Chapter 8)<br>• Complete evaluation form<br>• Support your evaluation with examples |
| *Modified with permission: Langlois JP, Thach S. Evaluation using the GRADE strategy. Fam Med. 2001;33:158-60. |

## ❖ Preceptor Evaluation Form

*See "How Will You Be Evaluated?" on page 119.*

**Student Name** _____

**Preceptor Name** _____

**School or Program Sponsor** _____

**Date** _____

| *General Information* | *Yes* | *No* |
|---|---|---|
| 1. Did you feel that your preceptor's practice gave you adequate exposure to general internal medicine? | ❑ | ❑ |
| 2. Which of the following learner resources were available to you: | | |
|     a. Reference library | ❑ | ❑ |
|     b. Personal computer | ❑ | ❑ |
|     c. Audio-visual learning materials | ❑ | ❑ |
|     d. Self-instructional materials | ❑ | ❑ |
|     List materials not available that you feel would have been useful: _____ | | |
| 3. Did you routinely round with your preceptor in a hospital setting? | ❑ | ❑ |
| 4. How many patients did you have contact with per half-day session? _____ | | |
| 5. What was the degree of your responsibility concerning patient care? ❑ Too much ❑ Too little ❑ Appropriate | | |
| 6. How would you rate your level of supervision by the preceptor? ❑ Too much ❑ Too little ❑ Appropriate | | |
| 7. Would you recommend this experience to other students? | ❑ | ❑ |
| 8. Would you recommend your preceptor to other students? | ❑ | ❑ |
| 9. Did you achieve your educational objectives? Please comment: _____ | ❑ | ❑ |
| 10. Were your preceptor's activities consistent with your educational goals? | ❑ | ❑ |
| 11. Did your preceptor give you constructive feedback about your performance? | ❑ | ❑ |
| 12. Did your preceptor allow time for teaching-learning sessions (questions and answers)? | ❑ | ❑ |
| 13. Did your preceptor take time to review patient medical records? | ❑ | ❑ |
| 14. Did your preceptor take time to review patient treatment? | ❑ | ❑ |
| 15. Did your preceptor check the accuracy of your history taking? | ❑ | ❑ |

*continued*

16. What additional comments do you have?

_____

_____

_____

17. What suggestions do you have that would increase interest in and/or improve this program?

_____

_____

_____

# APPENDIX C

## Resources for Preceptors

## ❖ Commonly Offered Rewards for Precepting

*(See "What Are the Most Commonly Offered Rewards for Community-Based Teaching?" on page 10)*

### Enhanced Capitation

One potential economic benefit is a higher capitation rate for participating physicians negotiated on their behalf by the training institution. Some programs have negotiated 1% increases (Grayson MS et al. Promoting institutional change to encourage primary care. Acad Med. 1999;74:S9-15).

### CME Credits for Community-Based Teaching

Although most teaching programs do not qualify for category 1 CME credits, category 2 credits can be claimed by preceptors. Medical school and residency program administrators can send letters confirming and documenting your participation.

### CME Discounts

Participating in an institution's community-based teaching program may qualify the preceptor for discounts on CME programs, including conferences and printed, electronic, and Web-based products. Some programs may be willing to audiotape their grand rounds and make them available at no charge so preceptors can earn CME credit when it is more convenient to participate.

### Internet and E-mail

Many programs have the capability to connect their community-based office practices to the Internet, thus allowing the preceptor and learner access to literature-retrieval databases (e.g., MEDLINE), e-mail, the institution's health care database, and teaching resources. As a further incentive, tutorials on how to use these various programs and services can be provided by the sponsoring institution.

### Textbooks

Textbooks can be provided to some office sites by the sponsoring institution.

### Recognition Dinners

Annual receptions or dinners recognize the volunteer efforts of the preceptors are a popular method of distributing preceptor awards. These events can be used to hand out either teaching awards or recognition certificates.

### Certificates of Appreciation

Most local programs offer certificates or letters of appreciation.

## ❖ Faculty Development Resources for Preceptors

*(See "Are There Courses To Improve Your Teaching?" on page 12 in Chapter 1)*

### Faculty Development Programs

Some institutions and professional societies offer faculty development programs for their preceptors. For a listing of available faculty development workshops or resources near you, call the Department of Continuing Medical Education at your local hospital, medical school, or professional society. Faculty development resources can also be identified by searching the Internet. On your web browser enter the search terms "Faculty Development" AND >your specialty<. For example, to search for faculty development resources in internal medicine enter "faculty development" AND "internal medicine." The Teaching in Your Office Electronic Enhancement also contains links to selected faculty development programs www.acponline.org/acp_press/teaching_in_your_office.

### Teaching in Your Office Electronic Enhancement

This textbook is associated with a collection of paper tools (forms, checklists, surveys) than can be downloaded, printed, and used in your office to help you teach students and residents. This site also contains links to other helpful internet resources to help you improve your teaching, such as faculty development programs, assessment tools, training competencies, tips on evaluating the medical literature, and teaching evidence-based medicine. See www.acponline.org/acp_press/teaching_in_your_office.

# Index

practice phase of, 93
skill checklist for, 89-90
unconscious awareness of, 88
Professionalism
as core competency, 18
teaching of, 20, 22

**Q**

Quality of supervision, 3-4
Questioning
in Microskills model, 54-56
preprogrammed answers to, 71

**R**

Rating of learning experience, 7
Receptionist
to inform patients about learner, 35
in preparation for learner, 26
Reflection
in case-based learning, 68-69
in teacher evaluation, 120-121
Reinforcement, 57-58
Reporter in RIME evaluation, 111, 112, 115
Resident, documentation requirements for, 36
Resources for faculty development, 121-122
Responsibility
of learner, 29
meaningful, 39-40
Rewards for community-based teaching, 10
RIME evaluation framework, 112-115
Role model
of behavior, 43-44
desired characteristics of, 41
Role of preceptor, 6
Room presentation, 76-78
Rules
general, 56-57
for Medicare documentation, 37-38
telling student about, 29

**S**

Satisfaction, student, 4
Scheduling
of evaluation, 116
of feedback, 99-100
patient, 29, 31-34
Script for office visit, 46-47
Selection of patients, 44-45
Self-assessment, 101-102
Self-directed learning, 82-84
Service-based education, 81-82
Shave biopsy checklist, 90

Site visit, peer, 122
Skill checklist, 89-90
Skills, teaching of, 39-49
meaningful responsibility and, 39-40
patient selection for, 44-45
strategies for, 45-48
teacher characteristics for, 40-44
SNAPPS model, 66-68
Stimulating learner interest, 41
Student. *See* Learner
Summative evaluation, 106
Supervision, quality of, 3-4
Supporting evidence, probing for, 54-56
Systems-based practice
as core competency, 19
teaching of, 21, 22

**T**

Teacher
benefits to, 9-10
concerns of, 8
desired characteristics of, 40-44
evaluation of, 119-122
office-based, availability of, 2-3
Teacher development, 12
Teacher-centered teaching, 69-71
Teaching. *See also* Community-based teaching
about ancillary procedures, 34-35
dual, 80-81
efficient, 75-85
goals of, 19-22
of interpersonal and communication skills, 20, 21
of medical knowledge, 19, 20, 21
method of, 29-30
of patient care, 19
of practice-based learning and improvement, 20, 21
preparation for, 25-38. *See also* Preparation for teaching
of procedures, 87-95
of skills, 39-49
of systems-based practice, 21, 22
Teaching experience, 11
Teaching points, number of, 43

**V**

Value-added benefit, 9-10
Visit, peer site, 122

**W**

Wave schedule, 31-34
Workshops for preceptors, 121
Workspace, telling learner about, 30